OVERCOMING ADDICTION

OVERCOMING ADDICTION

Seven Imperfect Solutions and the End of America's Greatest Epidemic

Gregory E. Pence

ROWMAN & LITTLEFIELD
Lanham • Boulder • New York • London

Published by Rowman & Littlefield
An imprint of The Rowman & Littlefield Publishing Group, Inc.
4501 Forbes Boulevard, Suite 200, Lanham, Maryland 20706
www.rowman.com

6 Tinworth Street, London SE11 5AL, United Kingdom

British Library Cataloguing in Publication Information Available

Library of Congress Cataloging-in-Publication Data

Names: Pence, Gregory E., author.
Title: Overcoming addiction : seven imperfect solutions and the end of America's greatest epidemic / Gregory E. Pence.
Description: Lanham : Rowman & Littlefield Publishing Group, [2020] | Includes bibliographical references and index. | Summary: "Leading bioethicist Gregory Pence demystifies seven foundational theories of addiction to reveal how they must work together to build more comprehensive solutions. Concerned citizens, individuals suffering from addiction, their families, and those who devote their lives to fighting addiction will find this new perspective a hopeful call to arms"—Provided by publisher.
Identifiers: LCCN 2019042442 (print) | LCCN 2019042443 (ebook) | ISBN 9781538135037 cloth ; alk. paper | ISBN 9781538135044 epub
Subjects: MESH: Substance-Related Disorders—psychology | Substance-Related Disorders—therapy | Substance Abuse Treatment Centers—ethics | Addiction Medicine—ethics | Choice Behavior—ethics | Bioethical Issues | Models, Theoretical | United States
Classification: LCC RC564 (print) | LCC RC564 (ebook) | NLM WM 270 | DDC 362.29—dc23
LC record available at https://lccn.loc.gov/2019042442
LC ebook record available at https://lccn.loc.gov/2019042443

♾ ™ The paper used in this publication meets the minimum requirements of American National Standard for Information Sciences—Permanence of Paper for Printed Library Materials, ANSI/NISO Z39.48–1992.

CONTENTS

PREFACE

> If I had to say where my drinking began, which *first time* began it, I might say it started with my first blackout, or maybe the first time I sought blackout, the first time I wanted to be absent from my own life. Maybe it started the first time I threw up from drinking, the first time I dreamed about drinking, the first time I lied about drinking, the first time I dreamed about lying about drinking, when the craving had gotten so deep there wasn't much of me that wasn't committed to either serving or fighting it.
>
> —Leslie Jamison, *The Recovering: Intoxication and Its Aftermath* (2018)

Almost every day, newspapers and other media describe deaths from drug overdoses. Preventing such overdoses raises some of the most pressing questions of our times: What causes addiction and its twin, alcoholism? How should they be treated? How much is the user responsible for his actions? Can victims overcome these conditions? What kind of society hinders, or encourages, abuse of such substances? As I shall argue, such questions raise not only factual issues but also philosophic ones. This preface sketches the issues discussed in this book.

In 2016, Surgeon General Vivek Murthy, MD, writing in the *New England Journal of Medicine*, bemoaned "America's escalating opioid epidemic [where] more than 2 million people in the United States are addicted to prescription opioids [and where] we estimate that more than 1 million people who need treatment lack access to it."[1]

In the western Canadian province of British Columbia between 2016 and 2018, more than thirty-eight hundred people died of drug overdoses. Worldwide, addiction and alcoholism are on the rise. In India and China, increasing amounts of alcohol are consumed per person year after year. In the Czech Republic, the average male over age fifteen drinks fifteen hundred beers annually, averaging more than four beers a day, every day, all year long.[2] Equally astonishing rates hold in Moldova. In Ireland, nearly half of pregnant women admit to binge drinking during pregnancy.[3]

In America, although the absolute amount of alcohol consumed per person has declined—mainly due to light beer and increased concerns about wellness—the amount of binge drinking has soared, especially in people under thirty-five. Sadly, as many as one in three extended families has a member with severe alcoholism.

As the number of deaths grows each year from alcoholism and overdoses of opiates, various experts claim to have discovered the true cause of both problems, as well as the only way to treat them. They write books, start residential treatment centers, and charge hefty fees. Starting with Alcoholics Anonymous (AA) in 1935 and ending with recent insights from brain imaging, counselors make conflicting claims about both ending alcoholism and treating addiction.

In this noise, we need to understand the foundational commitments of researchers and counselors. Just hearing one scientist pitch her views without opposing comments from others dooms us to incomplete comprehension. Getting to the truth about addiction and alcoholism requires philosophical acumen as well as hard-nosed facts. Getting to the bottom of the matter requires exposing the hidden ethical issues about treating addiction, such as how Google profits every time a desperate parent clicks on its misleading ads for rehab centers. Getting to the truth matters, not only to the people affected and their families but also to the lawmakers and taxpayers who pay for the cost of substance abuse and its treatment.

Take the bitter debate that occurred over treating addiction in 2018 in the normally staid *New England Journal of Medicine*. One famous neuroscience researcher claimed that addiction should be seen entirely as an "acquired disease of the brain." An opposing researcher in psychology found this view simplistic and countered that addiction was learned bad behavior that needed counseling to change.

Both of these opposing models thought that Alcoholics Anonymous/Narcotics Anonymous (AA/NA) used outdated and unproven methods. Moreover, the neuroscientist, psychologist, and AA advocates all believe that the views of ordinary people about addiction and alcoholism—as a series of free choices for which people are responsible—are primitive. Yet many people continue to believe that their loved one freely chooses to drink or inject. Are they all really so mistaken?

This book discusses seven models of addiction: Alcoholics/Narcotics Anonymous, Neuroscience, Responsible Choice ("Kantian"), Genetics, Coping, Harm Reduction, and Social Justice. Three introductory chapters sketch the history and nature of our epidemic, contrasting models of alcoholism and addiction, and money and treatment. Seven core chapters, each covering one model, follow the three introductory chapters. As the book progresses, each model is subjected to criticisms by both me and other models.

I start with the most famous model, Alcoholics/Narcotics Anonymous, and then progress to the latest model, Neuroscience. After those two, I discuss the other more traditional models. In each chapter on a specific model, I conclude by summarizing the model's explanation of addiction, its proposed cure or treatment, its explanation of why other models are mistaken, its view of whether addicts are responsible for their behavior, and its advice for families of affected relatives.

In a concluding chapter, I suggest avenues for further inquiry and my personal conclusions. In the penultimate chapter, I suggest that recent legalization of potent, recreational marijuana might create new crises of addiction.

These days, writing a book about alcoholism or addiction seems to require that the author be in recovery.[4] A companion view is that unless you've treated people for addiction or alcoholism, you can't write about it. Yet most writers in recovery write about addiction from the perspective of a particular model. The same applies for most counselors. The valuable passion of these writers often narrows their focus to the model that worked for them, making them ignore other models that work for other people.

This is an important point. If addiction and alcoholism are not all-or-nothing conditions, but rather spectrums, and if different people become addicted or alcoholic in different ways, then a one-size model won't fit all. These days, tolerance of other views is a rare virtue, but some prominent agencies are changing: The National Institute on Drug Abuse recently adopted the principle that "No single treatment is appropriate for everyone."[5] That's good and should be considered progress.

The literature and studies of alcoholism and addiction are vast, encompassing dozens of journals in many different fields. I have not read all these studies: I don't see how anyone could. But I have discovered the *philosophical assumptions* that emerge from this literature and how various models conflict with each other.

One thing I've discovered in researching this book is that almost everybody knows someone who's been in rehab for alcohol or drugs. Most of the time, their families don't discuss it because they're ashamed. However, once the news is out, they're eager to talk.

I've also discovered that discussing the evidence for or against various models is a touchy subject for many professionals, who often have a stake in the model of their home field. The same goes for families that have paid for rehab for a relative who successfully used a certain model.

For better or worse, I am neither an alcoholic, addicted person nor recovering from alcoholism or addiction. I have never treated anyone in therapy who is addicted or a heavy drinker. I have no monetary or personal stake in any model described in this book. Does that mean I can't write about these subjects?

My most general answer is that for the past fifty years, bioethicists have contributed immensely to intellectual life. Although they themselves do not perform abortions, assist patients in dying, or experiment on animals or people, they have discussed important ethical issues about all these topics. Just because you haven't performed heart surgery doesn't mean that you can't say something about the ethics of heart surgery. Similarly, just because you haven't treated people with addictions doesn't mean that you can't raise ethical issues about how people with addictions are treated.

Ideally, the people affected need an impartial survey of all models and their strengths and weaknesses. In that way, each person can decide which model, or which combination of models, works best for him- or herself or that person's child or patient. Thus, I believe that an impartial analysis can be valuable and add understanding to the issues.

AUTHOR'S NOTE

Like many who've studied these conditions, I believe that alcoholism is a kind of addiction. Although addiction is a broader category, in what follows I discuss these two conditions together. This may be a mistake, but if so, it is my mistake, and to prove it would take another book. I understand that some think the craving of someone dependent on opioids may exceed that of someone craving alcohol, but, as I will argue, the various *models* that try to explain these cravings and how to treat them say similar things about responsibility, best treatment, and reimbursement.

Second, in medicine and bioethics, we now urge everyone to use person-centered language, such as a "person with schizophrenia" or "a person with diabetes," not "the schizophrenic or "that diabetic." More important to this book, words such as *addict* and *alcoholic* carry horrible connotations and call up terrible stereotypes. These words, like the word *clone*, beg many questions.

"Opium" refers to the actual sap from poppies, "opiate" refers to a derivative of the sap that isn't the sap itself, and "opioid" refers to partially or completely synthetic agent that binds to opioid receptors. In this book, I follow psychology and neuroscience and use "opioids" and "opiates" interchangeably.

In general, I have tried to avoid pejorative terms such as "addict" or "alcoholic" and to use the more cumbersome "person with alcoholism," "heavy drinker," or "person with alcohol abuse disorder." At times, this makes for clunky writing, but I try to make up for it.

ACKNOWLEDGMENTS

The idea for this book actually came many years ago. I had long admired the late Herbert Fingarette, a philosopher in Southern California whose book *Heavy Drinking: The Myth of Alcoholism as a Disease* I had assigned in several of courses. After I wrote an op-ed for the *Birmingham News* on the ethics of treating alcoholism, and after I received both praise and abuse, I contacted Fingarette because I knew he had endured similar reactions. We started to correspond, and he sent me some of his books. He also encouraged this book.

I then wrote a chapter on the ethical issues of treating alcoholism for the eighth edition of my *Medical Ethics* textbook in 2016, and it proved popular. After that, I did my first podcast with Francis Sweeny, MD, host of the popular podcast *Straight Talk, MD*, on alcoholism and addiction, which proved so successful that it helped me think this book could be worthwhile and which led to several other podcasts with Sweeny on bioethics.

Alfred Garwood, one of my oldest friends from graduate school in philosophy at New York University and now an independent scholar, quickly read an early draft of this book and made helpful, encouraging suggestions. As a former library director and book publisher, his comments were very valuable at an early time.

Andrew Morgan, a visiting assistant professor in ethics at UAB from 2018 to 2020, very generously read every page of the first complete draft, making astute comments on each one. Vanessa Bentley, another visiting assistant professor at UAB during the same years, kindly improved my chapter on the Neuroscience model. Michael Sloane, a psychologist and neuroscientist at UAB who also directs our University Honors Program, likewise read that early draft and responded with eight pages of wise comments. Peter J. Hughes, a professor at the McWhorter School of Pharmacy at Samford University, also was helpful.

Daniel Hurst, a young bioethicist who worked for a year for a pharmaceutical company and who teaches bioethics for Cahaba Valley Health Care and our medical school and Honors College, also read an early draft of this book and made great suggestions.

Jason Gray, a young philosopher and ethicist who teaches at Auburn University at Montgomery and who taught at UAB for two years, wrote his doctoral thesis at UC Riverside on philosophical issues about addiction. I profited from reading that dissertation, as well as from Jason's extensive comments on the first half of a book draft.

During the first three months of 2019, I also had four research assistants from my Early Medical Student Acceptance Program: Hamad Muhmmad, Wendy Jiang, Victoria Chen, and Melissa Ebeling. Later, both Victoria Chen and Melissa Ebeling went far beyond what normal student assistants do and took "research assistant" to a new level. I am very lucky to have such brilliant, hardworking, careful assistants who will one day soon make great physicians.

Thanks to Kaitlin Burge and Matthew Hudson for assistance with the index and Carly Snidow for her astute proofing.

Although I began thinking about this book long ago, I finished it during the first months of 2019 while on my first sabbatical in thirty-two years. After chairing the philosophy department for six years, I needed to step away to finish this book. I am grateful for UAB for giving me a paid sabbatical, an increasingly rare privilege in today's academia.

Finally, I talked to many people who are dealing with having someone they love battle alcoholism or addiction. I also talked with some people who have recovered. As desired, I have kept them anonymous, but I am still grateful to them for sharing their pain and successes with me. Their stories and needs kept this book painfully real.

AMERICA'S UNSOLVED EPIDEMIC

> Heroin was different. I loved it. It was the first thing that
> worked. It took away every scrap of hurt that I had inside of
> me. When I think of heroin now, it is like remembering a
> person I met and loved intensely. A person I know I must
> live without.
>
> —Cheryl Strayed, "Heroin/e,"
> *Best American Essays 2000*

The numbers in the headlines each week stun us: In the year 2000, twenty thousand Americans died of drug overdoses, which seems like a lot, but just four years later, that number jumped to sixty-four thousand, implying that sixty-four thousand American families went through hell, often spiraling downward into financial disaster, sometimes accompanied by screaming matches about blame, and occasionally resulting in interventions that produced much resistance.

In North America and across the globe, the problems worsen each year. According to the National Center for Health Statistics, more Americans died in 2017 of drug overdoses than died from guns, HIV/AIDS, or car crashes—more than seventy thousand people.[1] Another study estimates that *every day* in 2018, between 174 and 200 Americans died of drug overdoses.[2] The search by journalists for good news became so bleak that their best hope in 2017 was that we had finally peaked at seventy thousand deaths in that year and that somehow, someway, that number would afterward ratchet down.

And so it was that, in late summer of 2019, when the Centers for Disease Control (CDC) had finally tabulated the tally of deaths from opioids during

2018, and after billions of new dollars spent on prevention and treatment, a weird hallelujah chorus erupted from America's media that the overall number of deaths had finally dropped a bit. The good news? In 2018, "only" 68,577 Americans died from drug overdoses.[3] The bad news? Between 2008 and 2018, at least four hundred thousand people in North America died of drug overdoses and perhaps three million were still addicted.[4] At this rate of "success," by 2025 the rate will be down to sixty thousand and "only" four hundred thousand more Americans will have died.

Opioids now cause the most deaths among Americans under fifty.[5] So many Americans died young that between 2015 and 2017 the overall average life-expectancy in America each year dropped.[6] We go "tsk tsk" when we hear that alcoholism in Russia each year has lowered the average life span, but a similar problem lies all around us.

But we've always had deaths from heroin and drug overdoses, right? Yes and no. First, since the FDA approved Oxycontin in 1995, two hundred thousand Americans have died of overdoses linked to prescription opioids such as Oxycontin.[7] Second, fentanyl is a new synthetic opioid, chemically designed as the ultimate pain-relief drug but fifty times more potent than heroin. To increase the effect, illegal drug makers weave fentanyl into heroin, cocaine, ecstasy (MDMA), and other drugs. In poor sections of some cities now, it is easier to get cheap, highly potent fentanyl than heroin. For people addicted to either fentanyl or heroin, lack of it causes misery, even suicide. Including alcohol in 2017, an astonishing one hundred fifty thousand Americans died from drug/alcohol overdose or suicide by overdose.[8]

By 2009, many millions of Americans had become addicted to oxycodone. When their prescriptions expired, they often switched to cheap heroin, which often came laced with fentanyl for the bigger high sought by addicted people. Eventually, as drug pushers and users sought better highs and more heroin contained fentanyl, thousands of users began to fatally overdose.

PROBLEMS OF DEFINING ADDICTION

Almost all definitions of addiction refer to both *physical* and *mental dependence* on alcohol or a narcotic, where users *feel compelled* to keep using and, when they try to stop, a *craving* to continue. When they do stop, they experience symptoms of *withdrawal*, usually unpleasant physical symptoms. At some point on the spectrum and as use of drugs continues, *tolerance* develops to alcohol, narcotics, and opiates, such that more of the drug is needed to get the same effect. At some point, habitual use becomes *dependence* and with tolerance becomes *addiction* and *abuse* of the substance. The term *substance abuse* is quite broad, covering abuse of opiates, alcohol, marijuana, legal and illegal drugs, and even psychedelic mushrooms.

In past usage, *addiction* referred to dependence only on substances such as alcohol and heroin, but in recent decades, the word has been expanded to include so-called *behavioral addictions*. A typical example is sex addiction, especially when people feel compelled to meet new dates for quick sex via social media; they admit that their behavior is not ideal, yet continue anyway.

Consider overeating as a kind of addiction, especially in the variety that produces body weights of six hundred pounds. We have recently learned from scientists (and science writer Gina Kolata[9]) that a 180-pound person who needs x number of calories per day to maintain his weight, and first gains and then loses an extra 100 pounds, his metabolic set-point at his newly restored 180-pound weight now requires fewer calories than x to maintain it. Metabolically, his cells are "screaming" for a return to 280 pounds, and if nothing is done to help him, he will probably give in and return to the larger weight.

Question: Is he at 280 pounds "addicted" to eating great amounts of food each day? On one hand, he seems to exhibit compulsive behavior that hurts his health and when he tries to eat less, he experiences a *craving* characteristic of people suffering from alcohol and opiate abuse. To help him resist such craving, neuroscientists claim he needs medications. As with alcohol and opiates, he might be genetically predisposed to being overweight, as well as need counseling about how to cope with stress without overeating. On the other hand, if being morbidly overweight is due to an addiction, then many "food addicts" exist in the world and millions more semi-food addicts. Conversely, whether one brings food to one's mouth seems paradigmatic of something over which one has control.

So, if overeaters have an addiction, they may have a disease that physicians should treat in clinics and hospitals. If overeaters have an addiction, then those who treat them should be reimbursed comparably to those who treat alcoholism and opiate addiction.

But how far can we take behavioral addiction? Consider *New York Times* columnist Kevin Rose, who picked up his smartphone 101 times a day and spent five hours and thirty-seven minutes a day on it. He went through "digital detox" with Catherine Price to "unbreak" his brain from his dependency on use of his smartphone.[10] Was Kevin "addicted" to using his smartphone? Did he really experience "withdrawal" like people addicted to opiates? Similar "cravings"?

Similarly, in 2019 the World Health Organization added "gaming disorder" to its International Statistical Classification of Diseases and Related Health Problems (ICD-11).[11] Addiction to video games now falls in the section of medical problems dealing with substance abuse and addictive behaviors, which includes "gambling disorder." Predictably, representatives of the video game industry criticized the move.

Yet the concept of addiction is vague: it has no sharp boundaries, especially in popular usage. At one extreme, every one of us with regular habits could be said to be "addicted" to our routines. At what point does a routine become compulsive? An addiction? At what point does "addiction" become meaningless?

Addiction's definition can also be political: Is a series of controlled, lifelong choices evidence of underlying addiction or merely a set of choices? Suppose an ex-smoker relapses every five years during a crisis and has a few cigarettes. In between, he does not smoke. Are his relapses evidence of an underlying, chronic, relapsing addiction, or does he just cope with extreme stress every few years by having a few cigarettes? The benign latter explanation differs dramatically from the negative associations of the first description of addiction.

"Addiction" thus has come to be used for so many different conditions that a common definition of it is hard to discover. All in all, the search for a tight definition of addiction, with necessary and sufficient conditions, may be futile.

Now let's go back in history a little. The drug substance opium, as well as morphine and codeine, comes from the opium poppy. This herb has always grown easily in places such as Afghanistan, where it has been cultivated by farmers for its high-cash value. These are natural products of the opium poppy that have been around for centuries. Drugs derived from opium are called "opioids" and the problem of addiction to opioids is ancient.

"Opioids" include prescription opioids, heroin, and synthetic opioids such as fentanyl. Common narcotic and opioid drugs include opium, heroin, codeine, oxycodone, hydrocodone, tramadol, morphine, hydromorphone, fentanyl, and carfentanil (a.k.a. "fentanyl for elephants").

DRUG COMPANIES AND THE MODERN OPIOID PROBLEM

Modern chemistry and drug companies have upped the potency of pain killers. The poppy plant is also the source of alkaloids that are chemically changed to create so-called *semisynthetic opioids* such as hydrocodone and oxycodone.

There are also completely synthetic opioids that bind to the same receptors in the brain as the above, such as methadone and fentanyl.[12] Fentanyl, fifty times more potent than heroin, is a completely synthetic opioid and the most dangerous of all known opioids because of its potency.

Of course, drug companies have been active in other ways to increase demand for their products. As bioethicist Carl Elliott writes in *Better Than Well*, Big Pharma wants to make us feel we need a pill to sleep, have sex, lose weight, or feel happy.[13] It wants to have our physicians prescribe Ritalin for our kids, Botox for our wrinkles, and Prozac for our moods. Modern man is awash in pills, and it is truly big business.

A new opioid epidemic started in America in 1995 when Purdue Pharma aggressively marketed its new drug, Oxycontin, for treating pain as a "fifth vital sign" and for treating perceived, widespread, untreated non-cancerous pain in patients.[14] This mattered greatly. Previously, potent narcotics such as fentanyl had largely been prescribed for unrelenting pain from cancer, but now the drug reps argued that many other kinds of pain, such as that from rheumatoid arthritis, post-accident injury to the spinal cord, and post–general surgery, should be treated aggressively with the new "safer" Oxycontin.

At the same time, pharmaceutical companies, especially Purdue Pharma, aggressively marketed Oxycontin (oxycodone) for pain to primary care physicians through their usual network of drug reps who gave physicians free lunches, expense-paid trips to vacation islands, and free samples. Critically for later lawsuits, drug reps largely dismissed the addictive potential of oxycodone.

Between 2000 and 2012, physicians freely prescribed opioids. The *Pharmaceutical Journal* notes, "Between 1996 and 2012, Oxycontin sales increased from US$48m to over US$2.4bn."[15] The same source states that between 1991 and 2009, prescriptions for opioids increased 300 percent in America and, amazingly, 850 percent in Canada.

By 2009, Purdue Pharma and the British firm Indivior pushed a few high-prescribing physicians to double their output, urging them to write more prescriptions and at higher, more profitable dosages, all the while urging their drug representatives to assure physicians that prescriptions for oxycodone or fentanyl did not create addicted patients.[16] In the same year, the United States consumed 99 percent of the world's hydrocodone and 81 percent of its oxycodone.[17]

In 2018, the attorney general of Massachusetts sued Purdue Pharma and the Sackler family for pushing oxycodone on patients when they knew how dangerous their drugs were. Some of the documents discovered by the attorney general showed Richard Sackler pushing sales reps to blame patients for their addictions: "We have to hammer on the abusers in every way possible," he wrote in 2001. "They are the culprits and the problem. They are reckless criminals."[18] This is the classic strategy of blaming the victim, as with the man who physically abuses his wife and claims that she is to blame because she isn't more agreeable.

By May 2019, attorney generals in forty-five states, as well as two thousand local and tribal governments, were suing Purdue Pharma and Insys Pharmaceuticals (makers of Subsys, a form of fentanyl sprayed on the tongue) and their distributors.[19] Juries agreed, returning verdicts against Insys executives. Insys agreed to pay $225 million in fines in Massachusetts for misleading physicians and patients.[20]

The Sackler family owned much of Purdue Pharma, made billions, and for years gave lavishly to charity. In 2019, activists chained themselves to the railings of the Guggenheim Museum to protest gifts earned from sales of Oxycontin.[21] Subsequently, the Metropolitan Museum of Art in New York declined to accept any more "Oxy-cash" from this family.[22]

Overdoses of illegal, imported fentanyl in 2018 killed the most Americans, a drug so dangerous that first responders wear Nitrile gloves in treating victims of overdoses.[23] If first responders mistakenly get a few salt-sized grains on their hands, other first responders rush them to emergency rooms.

Much of this illegal fentanyl originally came from China. So far, authorities have not been able to stem the massive, continuing smuggling of Chinese fentanyl into North America. This drug can be bought online from China and shipped by mail to almost anywhere, especially through the United States Postal Service, which has not been able to screen for fentanyl the way UPS and FedEx do.[24]

Some fentanyl also now comes from Mexico. In one bust at the US-Mexico border in 2019, in the false bottom of a large truck, agents seized 254 pounds of fentanyl (as well as 395 pounds of methamphetamine).[25] Fentanyl-laced oxycodone pills (a.k.a. "Mexican oxy") now flood across the US-Mexico border, spiking overdose deaths in Arizona.[26]

Although the number of prescriptions issued by physicians and dentists per person has dropped, many opioids are still prescribed. In 2012, about eighty opioid prescriptions were made for every one hundred Americans, and by 2017, that number had dropped to sixty opioid prescriptions per one hundred Americans.[27]

After an injury in sports, ordinary people get a prescription for opioids or narcotics. Some started down the road to addiction as adolescents when their wisdom teeth got pulled and they received narcotics. These patients liked the feeling and kept using the prescribed drugs. When the prescription ran out, they bought more on the black market or got another prescription. When these attempts ended, they turned to cheap, illegal alternatives, such as heroin.[28]

Nevertheless, the figure of sixty opioid prescriptions for every one hundred Americans is still high and far greater than it was two decades previously. Opioids from such prescriptions in 2017 in America still accounted for seventeen thousand overdose deaths—an agonizingly high number.[29] In 2019, federal prosecutors arrested thirty-one physicians between Cincinnati, Ohio, and rural Kentucky for illegally prescribing millions of prescriptions for opiates, sometimes prescribing them in return for sex.[30]

The *New York Times* estimates the number of addicted Americans in 2018 to be between eighteen and twenty-three million.[31] But no one needs the *New York Times* to tell us that many Americans regularly use opioids: All we need to do is watch ads on television for laxatives for "constipation caused by opiate usage." (So now we need drugs to lose weight, have sex, feel better, and poop?) Those ads cost tens of thousands of dollars. How many new prescriptions must be filled to recoup the costs of those ads? They continue because drug companies make money running them.

Behind the scenes and largely hidden in shame, hundreds of thousands of families scrimp to pay for treatment of addictions for their sons, daughters, brothers, and sisters. But are they paying for evidence-based treatments? Are they wasting their money? Could their children in their mid-thirties, without any treatment at all, just "mature out" of their bad habits?

THE ARTS AND ALCOHOLISM AND ADDICTION

In the extensive literature of writers and recovery addicts telling their stories, accounts of wallowing in one's own filth capture the attention of voyeuristic readers who revel in the depraved depths that someone else sank into. Many memoires of alcoholic writers show how they thought they needed to drink themselves to the bottom to have something to write about.

The first example of addiction literature (or "addict lit") came in 1821, when Thomas De Quincey made famous the phrase "opium eater" (*Confessions of an English Opium-Eater*).[32] Leslie Jamison, a writer and recovering alcoholic, describes the many memoirs alcoholic writers contributed to this peculiar canon and almost all are middle-class whites. The contrasting idea— that most people by their mid-thirties quit drugs or alcohol or learn to control their worst effects—is not dramatic enough for our Hemingways. So, writers don't write about how their best work came when they were sober. Nor do we hear about writers who are controlled drinkers, only drinking when their writing is finished.

Alas, popular culture fosters the idea that creative genius depends on ingesting large amounts of alcohol or drugs. The artist frequently degenerates or dies (Jack in *A Star is Born* or Freddy Mercury in real life).[33] But the underlying message is that you can't be a great artist unless you plumb the depths of addiction or alcohol abuse. Accepting that idea has cost many artists their lives: musicians Elvis Presley, Jimi Hendrix, Billie Holiday, Michael Jackson, Kurt Cobain, Amy Winehouse, Jim Morrison, Janis Joplin, Prince, Judy Garland, Whitney Houston, Dee Dee Ramone; writer Truman Capote; comedians John Belushi, Chris Farley, and Lenny Bruce; actors Philip Seymour Hoffman, River Phoenix, Cory Monteith, Marilyn Monroe, and Anna Nicole Smith.

ALCOHOLISM

Late in 2018, the CDC announced the shocking results of its groundbreaking study of binge drinking: Americans consume *seventeen billion* "binge drinks" a year, half by adults over age 35.[34] The same study found that one in six Americans, thirty-seven million people, binge drink at least once a week; when they do, they consume about seven drinks per binge. That is a staggering amount of drinking, and that fact contradicts the fairy tale that, after they leave college, young adults "age out" of binge drinking.

If anything, binge drinking seems to *increase* after college, usually at the end of work weeks. Drinking may even start on Thursday evenings, resulting in "hangover Fridays" (when drinkers get sober Sunday for the coming week). And alcoholism affects everyone, from the lowest worker to the richest child, from news anchor Elizabeth Vargas to comedian/actor Robin Williams, where every week some celebrity seems to check into rehab for alcoholism.

The CDC defined binge drinking for men as consuming five or more drinks in two hours. For women, it was defined as four or more drinks in two hours.

In 2014, the CDC modified its definitions about heavy drinking. Prior to 2013, the official *Diagnostic and Statistical Manual* (*DSM*) of the American Psychiatric Association distinguished between alcohol dependency and alcoholism. In 2013, it discarded these two terms in favor of three degrees of Alcohol Use Disorder (AUD): weak, moderate, and severe.[35]

The age-old problem of AUD seems to be getting worse. According to the

Vital Statistics of the Centers for Disease Control, excessive drinking caused eighty-eight thousand Americans to die each year between 2006 and 2010 and killed one in ten between the ages of twenty and sixty-four.[36]

In its 2004 Global Status Report on Alcohol, the World Health Organization estimates that two billion people every day consume alcoholic beverages and seventy-six million of them suffer from alcohol use disorder.[37] In other words, more people drink alcohol than ever before, and binge drinking everywhere has worsened.[38] The Social Justice model of alcoholism asks "Why?" What huge changes in the makeup of societies encourages such drinking?

We might also ask why the link between alcohol and cancer has been downplayed. While everyone knows that tobacco is linked to cancer, the statistics about alcohol and cancer are so rarely mentioned that they often come as a surprise. For example, a study published in 2019 found that women drinking one 750-milliliter bottle of wine each week had the same risk of cancer as those who smoked ten cigarettes a week.[39] A study in 2017 by cancer researchers revealed that 70 percent of Americans were ignorant of any link between alcohol and cancer.

MORE LETHAL CHANGES

By 2019, fentanyl had become so cheap to make and so easy to import into North America that it replaced heroin on the streets of many cities in North America. There was no longer a need to wait months for poppies to be harvested in Afghanistan or Mexico and then processed before being smuggled into North America. Fentanyl also makes more money for drug traffickers. In cities with high numbers of IV-drug users, such as Baltimore, by mid-2019 heroin was often hard to find, forcing users to buy fentanyl.[40]

Yet fentanyl was so much more powerful and quicker to hit that older users preferred heroin. Harm Reductionist volunteers on the streets urged addicted people to "go slow" with their injections because fentanyl hit so fast and big that sometimes people passed out before they could call for help. They also offered strips to test drugs for fentanyl (which were usually not employed because fentanyl was everywhere in everything, even things that looked like Percocet or Xanax).

Thus, the business of drug trafficking adapted, producing a more potent, more lethal product, making more money and putting even more people at risk of overdose.

OVERALL

A huge, stealth epidemic of opioid addiction has been building in North America for three decades, egged on by aggressive, deceptive marketing techniques of a few pharmaceutical companies, resulting in a shocking number of overdose deaths between 2015 and 2020. As leading physicians wrote in 2019 in the *New England Journal of Medicine*, "The human toll of opioid over prescription now represents one of the largest iatrogenic epidemics in history."[41] At the same time, binge drinking and alcohol use disorder are growing worldwide, especially among people under thirty-five. The causes, treatment, and issues raised by these problems are the subject of the rest of this book.

WHAT ARE WE GETTING WRONG?

> Here I was about to smoke crack cocaine for the first time.
> . . . In seconds, my brain exploded, and I fell to the floor
> on my knees. My heart felt as if it would explode with light,
> with love. Everything inside me became mixed up with
> everything around me, all fear disappeared, and only the
> rapture of light and love remained. Pure bliss. Ten orgasms
> packed into one.
>   "Oh God, oh-my-god," I whispered . . . to this new magi-
> cal god that I loved with a passion that exceeded anything I
> had ever experienced.
>
> —William Cope Moyers, *Broken:*
> *My Story of Addiction and Redemption*

M any people may believe that understanding addiction is simply a matter of understanding medical facts. They may believe that genetics, biology, or trauma in early childhood predispose people to substance abuse, such that one high, one drink, catapults the predisposed into compulsive attempts to regain that first "high." They may believe that if researchers knew enough biochemistry about alcoholism and addiction, they could find a simple, pharmacological way to cure both evils.

I think these beliefs are, at best, incomplete and, at worst, false. Instead, I think that views about addiction and its treatment illustrate opposing philosophical models. Failure to understand these models, and the competition between them for funding, impedes the important work of defeating our new epidemic of addiction. This chapter sketches some of the most important models of addiction and reveals some of the conflicts between them. It also describes the six key questions that every model tries to answer.

Consider the strange alliance between two seemingly opposite models of addiction: Alcoholics/Narcotics Anonymous (AA/NA) and Neuroscience. Although Alcoholics Anonymous refuses to allow impartial observers to evaluate its claims through controlled studies—a sine qua non of a reputable scientific study—it does agree with neuroscientists that alcoholics and addicts are in the grip of a *disease*. Both models agree that not just any disease grips these victims but one that takes over the lives of victims, destroying free will and wrecking families. Both models agree that when such powerful diseases control people, its victims cannot overcome their problems alone and need the help of twelve-step groups or professionals whose specialty is substance abuse.

In contrast, what I call the "Kantian" view of alcoholism and addiction believes that both of the above views are not merely mistaken but mistaken in a profound way. From the Kantian viewpoint, the models of AA and Neuroscience contradict human responsibility and how we hold people responsible for their actions each day.

This Kantian view sees addiction as stemming from continuous bad decisions by free, rational humans—decisions for which those humans ultimately should take responsibility. At any given time, those humans could evaluate the harm that using alcohol and drugs has done to them and their families and then try to alter their behavior. According to the Kantian model, both AA and Neuroscience ignore this power at the heart of real change: the ability to choose to behave otherwise and, more important, the powerful belief that one *can* so choose.

Not all statements about addiction constitute a model or are model laden, but some statements can only be understood as part of a model. To understand how these models work in our thinking about alcoholism and addiction, it's helpful to discuss what counts as a model. In the following chapters, I will demonstrate how each model answers at least six questions:

1. What causes alcoholism and addiction?
2. How are alcoholism and addiction cured?
3. Why are other models of addiction incorrect or misguided?
4. To what degree is the addicted/alcoholic person responsible for his or her condition?
5. How can relatives hurt or help?
6. How should those treating addiction be paid or funded?

Each of these questions is briefly discussed below, except the last, which is the subject of the next chapter.

QUESTIONS ABOUT THE UNDERLYING CAUSE
OF ADDICTION

Addiction must spring from somewhere. Not everyone is prone to it or to becoming an alcoholic. Not everyone who tries dangerous substances ends up dependent. Indeed, most who try alcohol or cocaine do not become problematic users. This is especially true with first-time users who begin after their mid-twenties. Why is that?

Each of the seven models supplies an answer. For Alcoholics Anonymous, the downward spiral may start with just one drink—a drink that famously makes the drinker feel better than ever. In the well-known picture painted by AA, that drink leads to another and then to another until, at some point, the drink is controlling the drinker. For AA and its sister Narcotics Anonymous, a dark river lies just beneath the surface of every person, and it is oh-so-easy to fall into that current, against which it's very hard to swim. Without calling on a Higher Power, confessing in a group of fellow lost souls, or getting help from a buddy, victims will drown.

In contrast, geneticists emphasize how the prevalence of alcoholism and addiction can be analyzed along certain well-known hereditary lines. Over several generations, some families exhibit a pattern of substance abuse. Genetics model adherents also think that certain ethnic groups (such as the Irish) are prone to alcoholism and addiction because of their inherited dispositions.

For Coping model theorists, learned behavior for dealing with loss, stress, and celebrations powerfully pull some into heavy drinking. In Western societies, watching football, getting married, celebrating after exams, and finishing a week of work are associated with drinking. For social scientists, these learned patterns of drinking explain alcoholism.

Recently, neurobiologists have made their own contribution with a startling new claim: Alcoholism and addiction are *acquired diseases of the brain*. Addiction in particular results from deep alterations in the structure of the brain, making it impossible for the affected person to change. For neurobiologists, mere counseling or willpower will not stem the torrent because victims of diseases of the brain cannot just choose not to continue abuse drugs and cannot learn a different behavior.

Where neurobiologists go inside the brain to explain addiction, champions of the Social Justice model go outside it and, indeed, outside people and outside societies. These theorists take the lofty view from ten thousand feet up and ask how the structure of societies encourages or discourages alcoholism and addiction. (A fancier name for this model might be Psychiatric Epidemiology.[1] However, because I want to emphasize the ethical frameworks of different structures in society vis-à-vis drinking and addiction, I call it "Social Justice.")

Finally, the Harm Reduction model addresses the answers of all rival models and defers answering the question "What causes addiction?" This model accepts that we may never know the true answer to that question. In the meantime (where "time" may be decades or centuries), it stresses helping people with alcoholism and addiction to reduce their associated problems.

HOW CAN ALCOHOLISM AND ADDICTION BE CURED?

Not only does every model claim an answer to the question of the cause of alcoholism and addiction, but each one also claims to have answers to the related question of how to cure these afflictions. The differences are seen most dramatically in how various centers for rehabilitation approach treatment.

For example, some centers exist that practice "tough love" while others are highly supportive ("soft love"); some operate from conservative religious orientations, while others are explicitly secular; some follow Alcoholics Anonymous and champion lifelong abstinence, while others encourage substituting less harmful drugs for dangerous ones (e.g., pot for heroin); some charge no fees, while others strive to maximize profits; some are inpatient treatments in hospitals or clinics, others are only outpatient; and, finally, some are run by local, solo operators and others by national chains.

WHAT ARE THE MISTAKES OF OTHER MODELS?

Given that models compete for the allegiance of health professionals treating addiction, it is not surprising that each model also explains how rival models get things wrong. Rehab centers often embody these claims and counterclaims. Most models claim far more than that rival models get the facts wrong.

For example, many models associated with scientists or AA/NA believe that the Kantian model is not only prescientific but also *anti-scientific*, especially regarding the idea that victims can recover through mere willpower and that falling into addiction or alcoholism is a kind of moral failure. The anti-Kantians think Kant wrongly asserts a mystical power of the will that doesn't exist, especially for alcoholics and addicts. In response, Kant's claim is that these models contradict themselves in assuming that substance abusers can change.

Where the Neuroscience model locates addiction as damage inside the brain, the Coping model sees a problem in learned behavior or family dynamics. Where one explanation is *internal* to the addicted person, the other is *external* to that person. For Neuroscience, the cause and treatment of addiction lies in things not accessible by consciousness. Neuroscience shares with the Genetics model the idea that the causes of addiction lie *hidden* inside or underneath personhood.

HOW MUCH IS PERSONAL RESPONSIBILITY A FACTOR?

One of the most famous issues in the history of philosophy has been free will, paralleled by its companion issues of personal responsibility and blame. Addiction makes resolution of such issues a national crisis, especially for families of those affected by chronic users, who are often told they should not blame their son because he has a medical disease. Few philosophers discuss the free will or responsibility of the addict or alcoholic.

Conflicting beliefs about personal responsibility for addiction are seen throughout the history of America's view of narcotics. For example, the "War on Drugs" pursued big jail sentences for dealers and drug kingpins, giving the United States more prisoners per capita than any other country in the world. However, this "lock 'em up" model was itself at war with medical models of addiction, which emphasized a three-branch model of prevention, treatment, and help with sustained recovery.

The various models of addiction and alcoholism cover the spectrum of personal responsibility. The Kantian model makes agents responsible for their addiction, whereas the Genetics model absolves them.

WHAT IS THE ROLE OF RELATIVES AND FAMILY?

In most cases of alcoholism and addiction, the truth is that there is not just one drinker, one addict, one patient, but rather two (or many): a partner, a sister, a mother, a coworker, an old friend, even a grandparent. Every heart-wrenching story of a death from addiction is told by someone hurt badly, often a relative (the saddest: teenagers struggling with addicted mothers).[2]

Partners and relatives struggle with whether they are codependent on the addicted person, unintentionally enabling the addiction and not helping in recovery. Partners and relatives struggle with questions about whether they caused the addiction and are often accused of being "enablers" or "codependent." Parents agonize about whether they should have raised their child differently, should have been more loving, or should have seen the early warning signs.

Relatives and families are often neglected when policy wonks think about programs to help alcoholics and addicts. It is not far-fetched to conceptualize addiction and alcoholism as a family disease.

As we shall see, each model tends to assign a different value to the role of family members. For example, if a model thinks family dynamics plays a big role in addiction, then obviously relatives and spouses will play a big role in causation and cure.

COMPARING MODELS

It might be thought that discussing ethical issues about alcoholism and addiction in terms of seven different models inevitably leads to negative judgments about all models, as if we are concluding that one model is as good as another or that all models are bunk. That is not true.

Some analogies may help. In studying the ethics of different models, we don't expect one model to crank out the right answer for thousands of different cases. Instead, each model is a tool for analysis, and each tool offers insights about different kinds of cases.

Perhaps a better analogy for models of addiction is to see them as different perspectives on a problem. For example, we can see a building from below, focusing on its concrete foundations down to bedrock; we can see it from inside, as its dwellers see it; we can see it from the rooftop looking down to the street; we can see it amid other buildings on the street and its relation to them; or, finally, we can see it from high overhead, the way Google Earth allows us to swoop down from above. None of these different views is best for all purposes, but each may be best for a particular purpose.

Of course, some models contradict or belittle other models. But if we put aside at the start the idea that any one of them captures the whole truth and nothing but the truth about addiction, then we will be more open minded about insights offered by any particular model.

CONCLUSION

The last question every model must answer concerns how those treating addiction should be paid or funded. Because it's so important and in the background of many models, that question will be discussed separately in the following chapter. Although money doesn't determine everything in bioethics or addiction, it should not be ignored.

In summary, every model tries to answer six big questions about alcoholism and addiction. They try to explain causes, best treatments, why other models go wrong or worsen the problem, how money should be spent (or not), how responsible the affected client/patient is, and what families should (or should not) do. The seven models are:

1. Alcoholics/Narcotics Anonymous ("a medical disease")
2. Neuroscience ("chemicals and electrical impulses")
3. Kantian ("poor choices")
4. Harm Reduction ("avoiding the worst outcomes")
5. Genetics ("written in the DNA")
6. Coping ("bad ways of coping")
7. Social Justice ("beyond the individual")

FOLLOW THE MONEY

It's such a savage thing, to lose your memory, but the crazy part is, it doesn't hurt one bit. A blackout doesn't sting, or stab, or leave a scar when it robs you. Close your eyes and open them again. That's what a blackout feels like. The blackout scattered whatever pixie dust still remained from the night before, and I was spooked by the lost time. I had no idea this could happen. You could be present and not there at all.

—Sarah Hepola, *Blackout: Remembering*
the Things I Drank to Forget

It is standard in bioethics to address monetary issues that affect outcomes. With alcoholism and addiction, only naive people would ignore the vast profits to be made by treating and studying addiction and alcoholism. This chapter describes the huge amounts of money at stake, how our present financial schemes have come to pass, and the ethical issues they raise.

Critics of the claims of various models urge readers to follow the money trail behind the success of the rehab industry and its claims about treating alcoholism and addiction. For example, critic Herbert Fingarette writes:

It is in the interest of the medical attack on alcoholism that large sums of money be reliably accessible to researchers and therapists. . . . Nor should one ignore the professional and financial stakes in what has become a rehabilitation industry employing many thousands of professionals and semi-professionals and generating many hundreds of millions in income.[1]

BACKGROUND

How did research in addiction medicine become so well funded? First, the Society for Neuroscience, founded in 1980, successfully lobbied Congress between 1980 and 2000 for increased appropriations for research about the brain. That research was funded through the National Institutes of Health and the National Institute of Mental Health. During this decade, the National Institute on Drug Abuse (NIDA) became part of the National Institutes of Health. In 1974, the National Institute on Alcohol Abuse and Alcoholism became a separate institute of NIH. It funds 90 percent of research on alcoholism. In the last decade, money poured into the organization. For example, its budget jumped from $458 million in 2013 to $2 billion in 2019.[2]

Next, President George W. Bush signed a federal law in 2008 requiring parity of coverage by insurance companies for both physical and mental diseases. In 2010, the Patient Protection and Affordable Care Act (a.k.a. "Obamacare") expanded coverage under Medicaid for treatment of alcoholism and addiction.

Under this new program, many states expanded Medicaid, the state-federal program that covers poor people, and thereby expanded coverage for treatment for addicted/alcoholic patients. By 2019, one in three people with opioid addictions could get treatment under Medicaid, providing an unintended boon to all addiction clinics.[3]

And the federal government feels pressure to spend more. In the last year of the Obama administration, $1 billion was allocated to states to fight addiction. In 2017, the Trump administration added another $1 billion. All of this added on top of $2 billion from the National Institute on Drug Abuse.[4] For Blue Cross Blue Shield, the number of claims has doubled since 2010 for treatment for opioid addiction for college-age patients.[5]

THE BUSINESS OF TREATING ALCOHOLISM AND ADDICTION

Treating addiction and alcoholism is a lucrative business. In 2017, rehabilitation centers for alcoholism and addiction earned *$35 billion*—an astonishing sum.[6] Families go broke paying for this treatment.

But how are we to know what to fund without understanding the strengths and weaknesses of different models? Should we fund models whose therapists refuse to submit results to impartial observers? Whose counselors cannot provide real evidence of success? If we throw gobs of money at scammers, won't that be wasteful?

Under the unique American system, most people do not pay for the true costs of their drugs. Drugs and treatment for addiction fall under group plans, so although we all pay for drugs and treatment through premiums and taxes, the real cost of these things is hidden from us. As long as our co-pays and deductibles are small, we don't complain.

Because so much money pours into treatment, rehab centers have proliferated. In 2017, the *New York Times* concluded that "the industry of addiction treatment is haphazardly regulated, poorly understood, and expanding at a rapid clip, bringing in $35 billion a year."[7]

In 2012, Michael Cartwright started American Addiction Centers (AAC), eager to cash in on the estimated twenty-three million Americans who had yet to get treatment. He intended to create a Mayo Clinic for addiction.[8] By 2018, AAC operated clinics in eight states, but in some cases Cartwright went too far, pressuring counselors to "close the sale" by admitting more new, insured patients, even threatening to fire counselors with low admissions.[9]

The amount of money such centers make defies belief. Inpatient centers can bill insurers $10,000 for twenty-eight days of service to an insured client. According to *Bloomberg News*, a single patient can generate hundreds of thousands of dollars in revenue, especially if we count rich patients.[10] Harvard Medical School's McLean Hospital, one of the premier hospitals in the world for treating alcoholism, addiction, and other psychiatric disorders, doesn't even take reimbursement and costs $50,000 a month.

By 2019, treatment for alcoholism and addiction in such centers had cost insurers *$35 billion*.[11] "Pill mills" in Florida have been described as the "gas on the fire" of the nation's opioid crisis, where, in 2010, ninety of the nation's top one hundred opioid prescribers were physicians in Florida.[12]

Florida also became the state with the most rehab centers, with more than fifteen hundred licensed facilities.[13] How much of the premiums paid by the average worker goes toward covering such treatment?

Our system allows some companies to game the system. Here's another issue: Few families know the difference between the fanciest, in-patient, residential center for treatment of addiction, which can cost $50,000 a month, and the much cheaper ones using the "Florida model." The Florida model has created a new way to makes lots of money.

Rehab centers based on this model have proliferated across the country. During the day, they rent offices for clients to attend group meetings or even work, but the clients sleep elsewhere at night in cheap group homes, often supervised by a person recovering from addiction.[14]

Some rehab centers in Florida or Prescott, Arizona, charge exorbitant fees for the daily testing of urine, $4,000 a test rather than the normal fee charged for elderly patients under Medicare ($200). To make matters worse, these centers test clients during the day when they work and test clients again at night when they sleep in a group home.[15] Why and how do they do that? They test twice and bill high because insurance companies reimburse them. The insurance companies then pass the costs along to everyone via higher premiums.

So, that's $8,000 a day for tests for each client in a rehab program! Some wits say that the cartridges that fill our home printers are "liquid gold" because they cost so much. But we now have a new candidate for that title.

In 2019, papers that were discovered under subpoena from the attorney generals of New York and Massachusetts against Purdue Pharma revealed a endeavor called Project Tango. In this project, Purdue executives proposed making money from the opioid epidemic in two different ways: first, on the front end, by aggressively pushing prescriptions for Oxycontin, and second, on the back end, by investing in centers that treated addiction for Oxycontin and other addictive drugs. One internal document from Purdue described how treatment of pain and addiction were naturally linked like a big blue funnel: "The fat end was labeled 'pain treatment'; the narrow end was labeled 'opioid addiction treatment.' "[16]

THE DARK SIDE OF GOOGLE

We should feel sorry for families of affected users. When a son or daughter decides to try to finally kick a habit, families lack the time and emotional strength to do research—the way they would before spending $40,000 for a new car or for a year at a private college. According to research by the *New York Times*, "More than 200,000 people seek addiction treatment on the phone or online every month."[17] That amazing statistic pulls back the curtain on the hidden agony affecting thousands of families, who sometimes attend public vigils at funerals of millennials slain by opiates, crying and holding signs that say, "Not one more!"[18]

Clients seeking recovery from alcohol or opioid dependency represent big money to rehab centers, as much as $40,000 over a few months. Few families know that Google auctions phrases such as "top rehab center for addiction." As a result, ads for shady clinics can appear at the top of its lists. Not every family notices the tiny green box that says "Ad" on the listing.

In 2018, Google took the extraordinary step of regulating ads by rehab centers. Why? Because a grand jury in Florida found the company guilty of selling ads to unscrupulous centers that gamed insurance companies for maximal profit.[19]

Google makes a lot of money selling these ads. According to *Bloomberg News*, a district attorney in Florida found that in 20,000-plus searches on Google for "drug rehab locations," Google made $187 per click on an ad for a center and $135 per click on "drug rehab centers and location."[20]

Those numbers sound impossibly high, right? How can it be worth it to rehab clinics to pay $187 per click? Well, consider if only one person enters the rehab clinic after one hundred people click on the ad. Those one hundred clicks cost the center $18,700. Reimbursement for one person's treatment can be $40,000, and if a new person is an extra client on top of the center's current clients and expenses, the center nets $21,300.

Of course, the centers that appear first on Google's list are not necessarily good centers by any criteria; they just paid the most for their ad to appear high on the list.

Few families also know that when they call the number in the ad (or respond to the "Chat Now?" box that appears when you visit the site), "lead generators" answer the phones—people who get a commission for referring a client to a center. Few know that when they call, they are put on hold for a few minutes while these "lead gens" quickly accumulate information about the caller's wealth, insurance, and desperation. With well-insured clients, these generators may even hold a quick auction of the client's business to competing centers.[21]

In late 2017, after criticisms from advocates for families of addicted people, Google stopped allowing the ads, mainly because they felt that the lead generators went too far. Less than a year later, Google again allowed such ads, but only for ones that (it said) had passed a certification test and did not use lead generators.[22]

THE OPIOID EPIDEMIC AND FIRST RESPONDERS

At the height of the opioid epidemic, or any epidemic for that matter, the burden on first responders is often overlooked and neglected. Whether part of an ambulance-based EMS agency or a fire/rescue department, all prehospital emergency care providers face a challenge greater than that of reviving and caring for an overdosed patient—that is, they struggle with burnout and compassion fatigue associated with repeated exposures to these types of calls.

Urban and rural first responders certainly don't share in any profits of the opioid crisis but must fund increased demand for their services. In two of the hardest-hit counties in Ohio, first responders may treat three to four overdoses a day, requiring two policemen, three EMS professionals, an ambulance, and interventionist drugs for each case. In the four years between 2014 and 2018, for just these two Ohio counties, their budgets for first responders, coroners, juvenile courts, the sheriff, public defenders, and preventive efforts increased by $20 million.[23]

In 2017, the Chicago Department of Public Health reported an average of twenty-one emergency responses (911 calls) to overdoses *per day*. For first responders having to run one or more overdoses every shift, this can have devastating effects on emotional and mental well-being. Moreover, oftentimes one crew will respond to the same overdose patient multiple times. It's easy to see, then, how this situation, combined with burnout, may affect how first responders view individuals who suffer from alcoholism and addiction. When a first responder must repeatedly respond and attend to a patient who is just as inebriated, "stoned," or overdosed as they were a couple days or weeks ago, it's easy to get frustrated and assume the mindset that the individual keeps making the same bad decisions that push them into a physiological state that requires emergency services (or that family/bystanders *assume* needs emergency services).

For this reason, one councilman of an Ohio city struck by the opioid epidemic proposed a "three-strikes" rule in 2017 to curb the rising expenses of providing emergency services to the community. In this policy, after responding twice to treat someone who had overdosed, 911 emergency centers would no longer respond if the same individual overdosed again. Although the councilman ultimately withdrew the proposal, it would be interesting to see whether this scare-tactic policy would simply result in more overdose deaths or if those who abuse alcohol and drugs would adapt and better manage their intake of those substances, thereby providing evidence of self-control and power over their supposedly uncontrollable disease.

CONCLUSIONS

All this information adds up to a national crisis of astounding dimensions. Coupled with massive debt from college loans, how can ordinary families cope with a daughter or son too dependent on alcohol or opiates? They need help, often fast, but how can the family know which model helps their child best?

It is too strong to claim that the way professionals are paid governs their philosophical views, but it is certainly true that most professionals who treat alcoholism and addiction are committed to one of the models described in this book. They may work for institutions that are similarly committed, making it difficult for them to try other models or to even think outside the box of their institution's framework. As the late philosopher Herbert Fingarette wrote, one advantage of being a philosopher studying these subjects, especially one who has done no funded studies himself about alcoholism or addiction, is not having a financial commitment because all the other "people involved in the (research) are all institutionally committed in some way."[24]

Not only does North America now suffer from an epidemic of addiction to narcotic drugs, but it also has a problem with a vast industry that profits handsomely from treating addiction. These problems piggy-back on our existing problems with treating alcoholism. Caught in the middle are patients and families, who struggle to find the best treatment and how to pay for it.

A MEDICAL DISEASE

Booze is a loan shark, someone [you] trusted for a while, came to count on, before it turned ugly. . . . Suddenly, you realize booze has moved in. He's in your kitchen. He's in your bedroom. He's at your dinner table, taking up two spaces, crowding out your loved ones. Before you know it, he starts waking you up in the middle of the night, booting you in the gut at quarter to four. You have friends over and he causes a scene. He starts showing you who's boss. Booze is now calling the shots.

—Ann Dowsett Johnston, *Drink: The Intimate Relationship between Women and Alcohol* (2013)

Since it began in 1935, Alcoholics Anonymous (AA) has become a famous model of overcoming alcoholism. Over time, a parallel organization evolved, Narcotics Anonymous (NA), and after the opioid epidemic began, NA became as popular as AA. In 2017, AA said it had more than 118,305 groups meeting daily in North America. In 2018, Narcotics Anonymous said it sponsored 70,000 meetings in 144 countries.

In the decades after the founding of Alcoholics Anonymous, it became a major force in politics, in funding, and in our culture. In 1944, it helped found the National Council on Alcoholism and Drug Dependence. Seven years later, the American Public Health Association gave it a Lasker Award for its contributions to public health. In 1970, it pushed for the "Comprehensive Alcohol Abuse and Alcoholism Prevention Treatment and Rehabilitation Act," which eventually led to today's National Institute on Alcohol Abuse and Alcoholism, part of the National Institutes of Health (NIH). In shaping these institutions, AA's view of alcoholism mattered greatly, especially its claim that alcoholism was a medical disease.

Founded in Akron, Ohio, by Bill Wilson and Bob Smith, Alcoholics Anonymous created a structured plan to help alcoholics recover control over their lives and to learn to live without alcohol. The name "Alcoholics Anonymous" came from an early book about the organization, *Alcoholics Anonymous: The Story of How More Than One Hundred Men Have Recovered from Alcoholism*, referred to by AA members as the *Big Book*.[1]

Both Alcoholics Anonymous and Narcotics Anonymous use a twelve-step approach for recovery. Indeed, their methods of using small groups of recovering alcoholics to help new members, of using the buddy system, and of using twelve steps for recovery are synonymous with these organizations, especially as they are portrayed in the mass media. Both have sister organizations, AA-Anon and NA-Anon, for friends and families of those affected.

Alcoholics Anonymous's emphasis on anonymity stems from the belief of its founders that its leaders should not seek personal fame, hierarchical power, or money from being part of AA. Although its twelve-step method has been adopted by many rehab centers (which may charge a great deal of money for their services), AA never charges people for its services—to its moral credit.

THE DISEASE MODEL OF ALCOHOLISM AND ADDICTION

The idea that alcoholism and addiction are not caused by upbringing, learned behavior, or psychological weakness, but by something deeply wrong with the person, has been around for a long time. In 1849, Swedish physician Magnus Huss first used the term "alcoholism" to describe a chronic, relapsing disease.[2] E. M. Jellinek, a researcher at Yale Medical School, famously championed the idea that alcoholism was a medical disease in the 1940s and 1950s. He worked closely for years with Alcoholics Anonymous (but later retracted his support).

James Milam, PhD, cofounded the National Association of Alcoholism Counselors and wrote a famous book in 1970 claiming that the life sciences agreed that alcoholism was a disease caused by genes, hormones, enzymes, and brain chemistry together working the wrong way.[3] Republished in 1983 and still in print in 2019, his book criticizes fellow counselors who believe that alcoholism is caused by cultural, psychological, and sociological factors and is therefore treatable through cognitive-behavioral therapy—that is, he criticizes what I call the Coping model in this book.[4]

By now, the AA/NA model has evolved into specific claims. Whether it's alcoholism or addiction, it claims that (1) some people—for whatever reasons—are susceptible to a specific, medical disease. This disease can remain dormant if vulnerable people never drink or never use drugs, but once people with this disease start using, (2) a specific pattern develops, one of inexorable descent to the bottom.

This pattern is the progressive nature of a disease with no easy cure, a downward cascade that can begin with just one drink or just one high. For most people, it begins with normal social drinking in high school or college.

For susceptible people—and this is a very important concept—drinking *becomes the central focus of their lives*. Eventually for heavy drinkers, every time they think about where to dine out, they think about which restaurants serve liquor. They only patronize places where they can get a buzz on before the meal comes. Their lives soon descend to the point where they cannot have sex, watch sports, or celebrate anniversaries without drinking or being tipsy.

This disease snowballs to blackouts, convictions for driving while intoxicated (DWIs), and loss of employment. Individuals keep using because (3) the pain of withdrawal makes them so miserable that they continue drinking, or using drugs, in part just to avoid the misery of withdrawal. With alcohol, this involves the so-called DTs of *delirium tremens*, which for most people includes heavy sweating, shaking, and muscular trembling; DTs may begin two to three days after cessation of drinking and may last two to three days. A similar three-day pattern occurs with withdrawal from heroin, but the symptoms there may be much more intense.

At some point in this descent to hell, according to the disease model, (4) victims lose all control over their drinking or their use of drugs. For this model, alcohol or opioids have now—to employ an oft-used verb—"hijacked" the victim's brain, making him merely a receptacle for the toxins pouring into his body each day.

For Alcoholics and Narcotics Anonymous, the diseases of alcoholism and addiction equalize down: they level distinctions of class, race, sex, celebrity, or income. Victims feel pulled by forces beyond their control. Victims continue atrociously bad behavior: hurting members of their families, stealing from old friends, or resorting to prostitution. The damage of this pattern escalates until (5) victims hit bottom, when they either die or desperately call on a Higher Power and others for help.

In Alcoholics Anonymous or Narcotics Anonymous, and for those seeking change, there is no negotiation with this furious, many-headed beast: the only path to salvation is lifelong abstinence, never having another drink. And there is no magic, no wonderous pill that erases the memories of happily being drunk, like those had by Frank McCourt's father in *Angela's Ashes*, who spent nights at an Irish pub, getting pass-out drunk while lustily singing songs with fellow drinkers, spending his paycheck, abandoning his wife and children to near starvation.[5]

TWELVE STEPS

One of AA's most famous methods is the necessity of following each of the twelve steps to recovery. As will be discussed in this chapter, the AA/NA model reflects a conservative Christian worldview about sin, atonement, forgiveness, and personal salvation. The twelve steps of AA's recovery program are as follows:

1. We admitted we were powerless over alcohol—that our lives had become unmanageable.
2. Came to believe that a Power greater than ourselves could restore us to sanity.
3. Made a decision to turn our will and our lives over to the care of God *as we understood Him.*
4. Made a searching and fearless moral inventory of ourselves.
5. Admitted to God, to ourselves, and to another human being the exact nature of our wrongs.
6. Were entirely ready to have God remove all these defects of character.
7. Humbly asked Him to remove our shortcomings.
8. Made a list of all persons we had harmed and became willing to make amends to them all.
9. Made direct amends to such people wherever possible, except when to do so would injure them or others.
10. Continued to take personal inventory and when we were wrong promptly admitted it.
11. Sought through prayer and meditation to improve our conscious contact with God *as we understood Him,* praying only for knowledge of His will for us and the power to carry that out.
12. Having had a spiritual awakening as the result of these steps, we tried to carry this message to alcoholics, and to practice these principles in all our affairs.[6]

The twelve steps of Narcotics Anonymous are very similar to the above.
Although twelve-step programs have been adopted by many rehab programs

around the world, it is not clear that scientific evidence supports them. This is partly because AA and NA do not allow empirical studies of their outcomes.

REMOVING STIGMA AND BLAME

When AA sees alcoholism as a disease, it may not actually be making a medical claim in the same way that physicians do—that is, it may not be saying that alcoholism is like cardiac myopathy, and it may not be saying that alcoholism occurs without any voluntary behavior. Indeed, it may recognize that, like lung cancer, the disease occurred in part because of previously chosen behavior. What AA and NA may be claiming is that, like an oncologist treating lung cancer caused by smoking, *blaming the alcoholic* doesn't help people stop drinking.

Claiming that "I have a disease over which I have no control" removes the speaker from the blame of others for his condition. "Yes," he might attest, "I voluntarily drank the first time, and many times after that, but at some point alcohol took over my brain and now I can't live without it: I no longer control it; it controls me." As one recovering addict, a college student, claims, "I wasn't a bad person. I was a sick person. Having a substance use disorder is like having diabetes or a heart condition."[7]

And it may be true that removing blame from the alcoholic or addicted person may help him recover. He may be ashamed of his past misdeeds: passing out in front of a daughter on prom night, losing a job, losing his driver's license, or, worse, killing someone while driving drunk. Even remembering these misdeeds may spur someone to get pass-out drunk.

HITTING BOTTOM

The concept of hitting bottom is another important, specific claim by AA and NA. It justifies the criminalization, discrimination, and humiliation of alcoholics and addicts. It supports tough-love models and making relatives feel guilty as codependent enablers. It has sometimes led to abusive methods in rehab centers.

Nevertheless, and as we shall see, it is far from clear that most drinkers hit bottom before they want to change. Nor is it clear that drinking alcohol always, or even usually, brings a progressive slide to the bottom. Finally, the claim that hitting rock bottom is the necessary, first step to recovery is highly disputed by other models of alcoholism.

THE RELIGIOUS ASSUMPTIONS OF AA/NA

One thing that secular models notice, such as models based in biological or social sciences, is that the AA/NA model is essentially Christian. Although AA has stopped making participants call on Jesus for help and now only mentions calling on a "Higher Power," the underlying framework illustrates long-standing themes of Christianity. In Christianity, the story of Adam and Eve represents original sin, meaning that humans are by nature prone to act immorally. The Fall of Man parallels the Fall of the Alcoholic or the Addict down to rock bottom.

At some point in this Christian theology, the wayward person critically examines her miserable life and realizes that she is lost, that she must ultimately confess that she has sinned terribly, and that she cannot reform herself alone. At this crucial moment, she must call upon Jesus and ask for forgiveness. After this existential moment, if she is inwardly sincere, she is born again in the eyes of Jesus and, for the first time in her life, becomes a true Christian. As such, her outer life moving forward exhibits her new inner bearings.

Over the centuries, organized Christianity formalized the confessional and added new conditions, such as Augustine's dictum that "There is no salvation outside the Church." Other people are necessary to be saved and stay saved. In a positive sense, the fellowship of a loving community lifts everyone up and keeps them from sin.

Going to an AA meeting and following its twelve steps sounds very much like having a true conversion experience in Christianity, especially because, in both cases, *no one else can do this for you* and only you really know whether you're faking. If you are faking, your behavior will soon show it, and fellow Christians (or ex-drinkers) will call you out.

More than the twelve steps, the *Big Book* of Alcoholics Anonymous makes it clear that its methods will not work with atheists and agnostics.[8] Take the story of Jim in chapter 3, who did everything in the steps except recognize a deity and his need to call on that deity for help.[9] For Jim, "All went well for a time, but he failed to enlarge his spiritual life," so he relapsed.[10]

Notice that this isn't just any Christian view: It's not the view of Roman Catholicism, Greek Orthodoxy, Episcopalians, Latter-day Saints, or Jehovah's Witnesses (and it's certainly not Judaism). It's the special brand of Protestant

Christianity associated with evangelism and proselytizing. That point is important, because if you weren't raised in that tradition, its methods may seem foreign to you.

This Christian worldview may resonate with some substance abusers, who may feel trapped by some dark force that feels satanic, who may believe in Jesus and the need for a new beginning, and who may need someone to forgive them for past sins. But for nonbelievers and non-Christians, it may turn them away.

CRITICISMS OF AA/NA BY HARM REDUCTIONISTS AND KANTIANS

Several well-known critics have long disputed all of the key claims made by AA and NA. The best known of these are addiction-physician Lance Dodes, philosopher Herbert Fingarette, psychologist Stanford Peele, and science journalist Maia Szalavitz. They might be classified as following the Kantian or Harm Reductionist model (or both). All of them publicized uncomfortable truths about AA/NA.

Poor Rates of Success

Perhaps the most telling criticism of AA concerns is its poor rate of success, a fact emphasized by Harm Reductionists. Although AA notoriously forbids controlled studies or external evaluators of its success, Lance Dodes, MD, a psychiatrist from Harvard Medical School who treated addicted people for three decades in California, estimates that of one hundred people who enter AA, only 5–10 percent kick alcohol for life, or about one in fifteen people.[11] That is not a very good rate, and nothing like what AA claims in its *Big Book*, which implies that anyone can follow its twelve steps and succeed (of course, AA can claim that those who don't succeed obviously haven't followed its twelve steps, but that is circular reasoning or else makes the claim unfalsifiable).

Data from *Alcoholism Treatment Quarterly* are even bleaker: Researchers analyzed AA membership surveys taken from 1968 through 1996. On average, 81 percent of newcomers stopped attending meetings within the first month. After ninety days, only 10 percent remained. That figure was halved after a full year.[12]

Suggestibility

The television show *South Park* has devoted several episodes to alcoholism; these episodes have been both popular and controversial. In general, the show's creators skewered the claim that alcoholics have a disease over which they lack control.

In "Bloody Mary," Randy drives drunk with his kids, gets arrested, loses his license, and must then attend AA meetings, which convince him that he has a fatal disease over which he has no control.[13] Because of his new belief that the drink-disease has him in her mighty grip, he drinks even more. In one controversial scene, everyone in his AA group agrees that they are powerless over their disease, adjourn, and rush to a bar.

As this episode illustrates, telling drinkers they have a disease may make them fatalistic and feel helpless. From the Kantian viewpoint, it makes them feel like robots.

A good deal of work in genetics and bioethics has concluded that presymptomatic testing for terrible genetic diseases is not good if the person tested cannot do anything to prevent the future disease. Critics of such testing, such as psychologist Nancy Wexler—herself at risk for inheriting Huntington's disease and who helped discover a presymptomatic test for this condition—warn that such testing might make a person develop a *sick identity* decades before symptoms appear; thus, a core part of a person's new self-concept is as a future sufferer of disease.

In the same way, putting the onerous label of "suffering from the disease of alcoholism" or "victim of addictive disease" on someone can alter his self-concept, making him feel fatalistic and creating feelings of hopelessness, which could even lead to more risky behavior because he thinks, "I'm fated to drink and die early, so I might as well enjoy myself."

Thus, applying the label "disease of alcoholism" on someone may relieve the stigma, but it may also relieve them of responsibility and allow them to be deceived into thinking they have no control over their drinking.

Adverse Selection

Psychiatrist Lance Dodes examined the few studies that tried to objectively evaluate AA's claims and found that only 5–8 percent of people who started groups were able to stay sober for more than a year.[14] He argues that the success of those who succeeded was due to adverse selection—that is, those who succeeded were motivated by AA's religiosity and all-or-nothing attitude.

Harm Reductionists think AA/NA works for 5–10 percent of heavy drinkers: those who think in black-or-white, all-or-nothing ways, the kind of person who believes that either he follows absolute, unchanging, absolute moral rules commanded by God or else everything is permitted (for example, either married with one, lifelong spouse or serial promiscuity). Such a person will either drink/inject to the maximum or not drink/inject at all. For him, no moderation is possible, no compromise.

The no-drinking-to-enter requirement also creates adverse selection into rehab programs, meaning only a small subset of drinkers or addicted people can be admitted. The many users who can't quit cold turkey cannot enter the program, even though they are the ones who may need help the most. Of course, if someone can't stop drinking, then she can't enter the program and can't later be counted as a failure. But then programs are treating only people who have already decided to change, raising the profound questions of whether these people could quit without the program because they (1) have finally decided to change and (2) found a way to begin being clean.

Loss of Control

Herbert Fingarette's examination of empirical studies about alcoholism led him to a startling conclusion: the majority of problem drinkers do not progress as the disease model predicts, instead learning to control their drinking and to moderate the ill effects of their drinking.[15] In Fingarette's terms, they become "heavy drinkers" but not "alcoholics"—at least not as the term "alcoholic" is understood by AA. Fingarette critiqued AA from a Kantian viewpoint, one emphasizing personal autonomy and self-control. He notes that "most of these programs, in spite of their loss-of-control doctrines, require the alcoholic to voluntarily cease drinking."[16] Not only do these programs assume that drinkers *can* choose to stop drinking on their own, but they also *require* it!

As Kant would argue, this argument is doubly contradictory, first in assuming people can choose to live differently, while claiming they are victims of a disease over which they have no control, and second in requiring people to have already quit before entering the program—a program that says they have a disease over which they have no control.

Even more threatening to both AA and the rehab industry in general, Fingarette discovered that most heavy users of alcohol, marijuana, cocaine, heroin, and opioids stop addictive behavior by their mid-thirties, that people learn to control their usage without total abstinence, and that people can learn to control their usage even without going to a residential treatment center.

Fingarette's article in the *Harvard Law Review* focused on the claim by AA/NA and genetics/neurobiology that drinking/using is *involuntary*.[17] He emphasized that, when pressed, lawyers pushing the disease model as an excuse for bad behavior by their alcoholic/addicted clients frequently hedge, moving from their clients having *no control* over their usage to *less* control than others.

The US Supreme Court in *Traynor v. Turnag* (1988) denied educational benefits to two veterans allegedly suffering from alcoholic disease. In its decision, it cited Fingarette and turned down the veterans.[18]

Fingarette notes that craving for alcohol was seen by some in the 1960s "as due to a destruction of certain centers in the brain, or as an involuntary, conditioned response to incipient withdrawal symptoms."[19] These "physical" models of alcoholism asserted that longtime drinking gradually changes the brain of the alcoholic. For all these reasons, lawyers for alcoholics in *Traynor v. Turnag* claimed that the continued drinking of their clients was involuntary.

In a neat move, Fingarette asked whether drinkers themselves believed that they could stop. Lawyers answered that their clients *did* believe that they could stop. Fingarette then cited numerous studies that show that most heavy drinkers can abstain or learn to control their drinking—facts that these lawyers found hard to explain.

In sum, Fingarette disputed four common themes about alcoholism-as-a-disease: (1) it unfolds the same way in all drinkers, (2) once the pattern of the disease starts, it is uncontrollable, (3) victims are no more responsible for their condition than epileptics, and (4) victims can only get better with the help of physicians.[20] Fingarette rejected all these claims, for which he was heavily attacked personally throughout his life.[21]

Lifetime Abstinence

The claim that it is okay to learn to become a moderate drinker, one essential to Harm Reduction, infuriated counselors and alumni of AA and NA. For them, the only standard of success in reducing the harms of addiction and alcoholism is complete abstinence for the rest of one's life. Any slip from this lofty ideal means failure. This is important because AA labels any heavy drinker who learns to moderate her drinking a failure.

This can set up a deadly cycle. If addiction and alcoholism are chronic, relapsing diseases, then few people will kick them for life. According to a 2019 survey in the *New England Journal of Medicine* about preventing opioid overdoses, "A prolonged period without opioid use (including methadone and buprenorphine) is both a sign of recovery and a risk factor for fatal overdose."[22] Addicted people who were imprisoned without treatment are at great risk for fatal overdose when they are released. Because of loss of tolerance during the drug-free period, resumption of old patterns of drug usage can kill them, especially if newer, more potent substances have crept into the market. In the view of the authors of this survey, the view of AA and NA, that abstinence is the only road to recovery and that using methadone or buprenorphine is a sign of weakness, merely replacing one drug with another, actually sets up patients for fatal overdoses.

Self-Deception of Alcoholics and Addicts

Finally, Fingarette offered one of the most fascinating, intriguing explanations for what occurs in the mind of all addicts. On his phenomenalistic account, all those addicted to alcohol, video games, overeating, sexual adventure, or cocaine engage in *self-deception*. Far from being a great puzzle about how heavy drinkers can deceive themselves, Fingarette thinks such deception is normal. Impulses or behavior that are shameful, or that produce guilt, pain us more when we focus attention on them.

Fingarette's view is illustrated in Caroline Knapp's memoir, *Drinking: A Love Affair*: "I looked like hell and somewhere inside I understood that if kept this up, kept drinking and working and flailing around like this, I'd die, slowly, but literally kill myself."[23]

Likewise, comedian Amy Dresner writes in *My Fair Junkie: A Memoir of Getting Dirty and Staying Clean*, "Substance abuse was unknown territory for me. I hadn't even ever been *around* drug addicts. I thought I was just a neutral tourist in druggyland, visiting, experimenting . . . even if that experimenting was all day every day. I was lying to myself, but I didn't realize it till years later. Or maybe I knew, but I wanted to believe the lies. Same difference."[24]

Fingarette wrote that when we divert our attention from shameful things about ourselves, they are less painful: self-deception allows us to distract ourselves from attending to what we find bad in ourselves. However, for Fingarette, "self-deception entails no special, aberrant, or otherwise distinctive mental maneuvers. It is a normal mental maneuver with the distinctive aim of avoiding acceptance of responsibility by means of deceiving oneself."[25]

This may be true and obvious. But if so, who's going to fund research into genetics or biology of alcoholism? This is not a view that can be used to secure funding or reimbursement for services in a rehab center.

Rock Bottom

According to its critics, who are legion, the claim that the addict or alcoholic must truly hit rock bottom may be the worst, most inhumane idea of AA or NA. Although this claim has almost no supporting evidence, the assumption that it is true permeates AA/NA, our court system, and popular television shows about addiction.

In essence, the rock-bottom claim seems to mirror the belief of slave trader John Newton, who wrote "Amazing Grace"—the idea of being irredeemably sordid and vile, without hope of salvation. In other words, it is a story of the Fall, of sinful behavior, and the only chance of salvation: a true, inner confession of powerlessness and need to call on Someone Else for help.

The rock-bottom claim indirectly denies that substance abuse can in any way be attributed to learning disorders or immaturity. If the Coping model is correct that (1) most people "mature out" of their immature behavior between ages fifteen and thirty, and (2) most of the above recover better with good jobs, supportive families, and good insurance, then the idea that people must hit rock bottom to recover, and especially to be *forced* to hit a rock bottom, is particularly pernicious. According to a literature review by William Miller and William White, "After four decades of research, in fact, not a single study has supported the confrontational model as superior to kinder and less potentially harmful treatments."[26]

Claiming that every addict must hit rock bottom before he truly recovers can be both circular and unfalsifiable in that if someone starts using again after rehab, it is claimed that they haven't really hit rock bottom. It can also be deadly: the one, undeniable form of hitting rock bottom is death by overdose or suicide.

Rock-bottom claims reinforce harsh prison sentences and lack of transitional or maintenance medication going into or leaving prison. If the Coping and the Harm Reduction models are the most humane models vis-à-vis alcoholism and addiction, confrontational techniques that force patients to hit a bottom are the harshest.

Philosophically, the intense moralism behind forcing people to hit rock-bottom directly contradicts the other major claim in AA/NA: that alcoholism and addiction are *medical diseases.* Oncologists don't force cancer patients to hit bottom before starting treatment, so what's going on with treating addiction?

Rock-bottom claims justify the idea of breaking people to help them reach rock bottom, so they thus justify abusive behavior by counselors and other group members in shouting down newbies, treating every heavy drinker and addicted person as a liar, manipulative, and selfish. Shows portraying family interventions, where the patient is ambushed in front of cameras, perpetuate the morality of these harsh techniques. Family members are criticized for "enabling" users and encouraged to use equally harsh, unforgiving techniques.

CRITICISMS OF AA BY NEUROSCIENCE

Neuroscientists both accept and reject the way Alcoholics Anonymous understands and treats alcoholism. Ditto for the way Narcotics Anonymous understands and treats addiction. The Neuroscience, Coping, and Harm Reduction models all agree that joining an AA/NA group and trying to follow their twelve steps are not enough for most addicts or most alcoholics to change. These substance users also need pharmacological help and the guidance of therapists and physicians.

Importantly, the work of neuroscientists fits the disease model in important ways that AA does not. Neuroscience fulfills some of the assumptions of a real medical model of disease.

A medical model's most important claim is that the cause of the aberration is not external to the patient in social or environmental factors but internal to his body, so to speak, "in his biology." Ideally, a medical model of alcoholism or addiction would specify the exact location of the area of the body or brain that has been affected, an area that presumably would be a target of experimental cures. Furthermore, the definition of the condition and its cure, whether alcoholism or addiction, would not be subjective but objectively verifiable by independent observers. This is something that AA has refused to allow.[27]

As we shall see, the claim about changes in the brain, either from drinking or from using opiates, is central to many models about the causes and treatment of alcoholism and addiction. It is the Holy Grail of either proof of a model or its failure.

Perhaps most important, AA/NA also doesn't say what to do about the physiological misery of withdrawal, other than to tough it out. That is a very hard road to travel, according to Neuroscience and Harm Reduction, which advocate substituting less addictive drugs and drugs that block the symptoms, such as methadone and buspirone. AA implicitly adopts the ancient Christian trope of "growth through suffering," but, as many critics of this doctrine have noted, some are called upon to suffer much more than others and sometimes the suffering doesn't stimulate growth but extinguishes it.

Spontaneous Remission

One of the most surprising findings in the literature of alcoholism and addiction postulates that addictive behavior commonly begins in adolescence, worsens in the twenties, and, by the mid-thirties, *runs its course when the brain or person matures*. In the slang of addictionologists, a lot of people simply "mature out" of binge drinking, being a pothead, snorting cocaine, or using heroin. Yet if the deep structure of their brain had been changed by a disease, this would seem to be impossible.

Borrowing a phrase from oncology, medical researchers have documented "spontaneous remission" among self-declared alcoholics and addicts, where the phrase is defined as people who quit using without any formal treatment. Lance Dodes emphasizes that the rate of spontaneous remission of heavy drinkers is important for determining a baseline regarding how many drinkers quit on their own.

Dodes found that each year after defining themselves as alcoholics, somewhere between 4 and 8 percent of drinkers simply stop drinking and remain sober for a year. Moreover, the numbers build over the years. A large meta-analysis published by researchers at Beth Israel Medical Center/Icahn Medical School in New York City concluded, "In sum, the preponderance of these studies suggests that a spontaneous remission rate of alcoholism of at least one-year duration is about 4–18 percent."[28]

A surprising number of heavy drinkers and addicted people "mature out" of this problem, regardless of the method used or, indeed, whether they use any method at all. As early as 1962, long-term studies based on data from the Federal Bureau of Narcotics showed that most adolescents were not ready to stop using, but that after 8.6 years, most addicted people had stopped using and would continue to stop for at least five years.[29] Although most people started alcoholic drinking or drug addiction as teenagers, by age thirty-five most had either gotten their drinking under control or stopped altogether.

Thirty-eight years later in 2000, a review of the literature of substance abuse revealed similar, if less dramatic, findings. Using a narrow definition of spontaneous remission from alcohol and hard drugs, 18 percent of users succeeded, and using a broad definition of spontaneous remission, it was 26 percent. Concerns about health and pressure from family helped create such remissions and changes of identity, family support, and different friends helped maintain it.[30]

Another study reached a conclusion that AA/NA would dispute: "Drug abuse . . . is not a terminal condition for most individuals."[31] The National Institute on Alcohol Abuse and Alcoholism funded a $27 million study to determine which program of treatment best matched the profile of an alcoholic person and came to the surprising conclusion that the best treatment only bettered no treatment by a 3 percent improvement in drinking outcomes.[32] Another study in 2005 by Dawson and colleagues found that in 4,422 male drinkers, after one year and where only 25 percent had received any treatment, 36 percent evolved to low-risk drinkers or abstinence.[33] A similar study came to a conclusion that both AA/NA and Fingarette would accept: that "drug abuse treatment is most effective [when] drug abusers are ready to change their behaviors."

MORE CRITICISMS OF AA FROM OTHER MODELS

A more general problem infects the AA/NA model here. The Social Justice and Coping models wonder about an expanding list of behaviors included in disease models of addiction. Nicotine in tobacco is addicting, but do smokers have a disease? What about gambling? Does repeated gambling constitute a medical disease? What about overeating? Is this also a disease? Promiscuous sex? Being on the internet all day? On social media? Can one really be a sex addict? More generally, does any semi-compulsive behavior qualify as an addiction and as a disease?

And what about the concept of addiction and personal responsibility? Either one has no need to make amends to others for wrongs done or one does. As we shall see in the chapter discussing the Kantian view, AA/NA seems to make the contradictory assumptions that the alcoholic/addict has a disease over which he has no control but also needs to apologize to people he previously harmed.

As for Harm Reductionists, they don't care what causes addiction or what helps someone kick it. They just want to reduce the most harm from the millions who use alcohol, marijuana, or narcotics every day. They aren't trying to make a new scientific discovery or find a permanent cure for alcoholism and addiction. In their view, we have had these problems for thousands of years and we will be unlikely to cure them in the next year or the next decade or maybe even the next century. In the meantime, we should focus on how to help users, their families, and the rest of society reduce the harms of usage.

Two final problems with AA: First, it purports to be endorsed by medical authorities but often cites only one physician. Of course, given the thousands of physicians who exist, almost anyone can find some physician, somewhere, to endorse any strange claim, or almost anyone can quote some physician out of context. Lance Dodes claims that from the beginning, the American Medical Association has been skeptical of AA and its methods.

Second, AA fails to mention a probable result emphasized by Dodes: Not only do fewer people improve in AA than the baseline of spontaneous remission, *but some people are also worse off after attending AA meetings*. Why? Because unless they achieve total abstinence for life, AA makes them feel like failures.

STRATEGIC VALUE?

Some counselors in AA or NA would argue that even if addicts don't have free will, telling addicts that they have free will and can quit is of great strategic value in therapy. In the same way, other counselors argue that even if alcoholism and addiction are not diseases the way most medical diseases are, treating them this way is strategically useful in many ways, especially in getting users into therapy, in getting insurance companies to pay for the treatment, and in getting funding for research.

One wonders whether a similar strategic model lies behind the push to classify more and more troublesome behaviors as addictions: gambling, over-eating, compulsive or promiscuous sex, pornography, computer usage, playing video games, and any kind of binge: alcohol, shopping, exercising, Netflix watching. If every addiction is a disease and eligible for medical treatment, then it makes sense to classify more and more problematic behaviors as addictions.

However, ethically and philosophically, there is a great problem with this kind of strategy: *it is a lie*. Lies by omission or diversion of focus already permeate the ways many corporations market themselves. How far do we want to go here?

If the truth is the enemy in treating problem drinkers, when is it going to be an ally? If counselors and researchers commit to such lies on the front end, how far down that deceptive road are they willing to go? Are we ready to buy into the idea that every problematic behavior is an addiction and a disease?

Are we willing to pay the billions it would cost to treat everyone with one of these addictions?

All this does not seem like an ethically defensible position. It also would waste lots of money.

CONCLUSIONS

AA and NA undoubtedly work for some people, especially those with a rigid, all-or-nothing personality and an evangelical Christian background. But the popularity of their methods belies the dismal facts that most people who try twelve-step groups fail to finish and that neither AA nor NA allow objective evaluations of their results.

Many other problems exist for these methods. First, by defining success only as lifelong abstinence, almost everyone who starts an AA or NA group is labeled a failure, which is unfortunate. Second, the worst cases of alcoholism or addiction will often need medication substitution to reduce the misery of withdrawal, which AA and NA oppose. Third, the assumption that changes can only begin after hitting rock bottom lends itself to abuse in rehab and harsh punishments in prison, for which there is little evidence of effectiveness. Finally, as I shall argue later, it is likely that the huge majority of people who eventually manage or quit their bad habits do so with a variety of techniques and may not need to be abstinent for life.

Summary of AA/NA

Underlying cause: A person suffers an inexorable disease over which he has lost control and which, alone and through willpower, he cannot control.

Treatment: The twelve-steps method, which has worked for millions of people, consists of confession in a group, abstinence for life, and, most important, personally letting a Higher Power guide a new life without alcohol or narcotics.

Other models: They make a major mistake in accepting moderated drinking, which true alcoholics cannot do. Similarly, substituting other drugs for alcohol or heroin, such as methadone or buspirone, is a mistake and just substitutes one addictive drug for another without any inner spiritual change in the user.

Responsibility: Alcoholics and addicts are victims and are not responsible for contracting their diseases; however, they are responsible for going to AA meetings, ceasing to drink, and calling buddies in crisis.

Family matters: AA and NA have separate groups for relatives and families of their members. Although relatives can do some things to help, unless the person affected decides to stop using, joins a group, and calls on a Higher Power, relatives can do little.

Money: Those helping addicted people and alcoholics recover should be volunteers—at least those working in Alcoholics and Narcotics Anonymous.

CHEMICALS AND ELECTRICAL IMPULSES

> After a summer of addiction to heroin, word started to get around that I was using heavily and that was bad for my career. I suddenly got the best offer of my life for my career and knew I had to stop. So, I went cold turkey for three days. What was that like? Imagine the worst flu you ever had and then imagine at the same time sticking your finger into a live, electrical socket. That's what it was like. It was hell and I never want to go through it again, and I never did.
>
> —Confession of a former heroin addict to the author

The interdisciplinary field of neuroscience has built a different model of addiction, one rooted in new discoveries about biology and the brain. Neuroscience consists of scientific researchers from many fields who focus on studies of the nervous system, especially neurons and how they communicate. Neuroscience came into its own in the second half of the twentieth century, especially between 1990 and 1999, a decade designated by President George H. W. Bush as the "Decade of the Brain."

Nora Volkow, MD, director of the National Institute on Drug Abuse, penned a crusading overview in 2016 about her view of addiction in the *New England Journal of Medicine*, where she wrote, "After centuries of efforts to reduce addiction and its related costs by punishing addictive behaviors failed to produce adequate results, recent basic and clinical research has provided clear evidence that addiction might be better considered and treated *as an acquired disease of the brain*" (emphasis added).[1]

Volkow's view is not new. Twenty years before, in 1997, psychologist Alan

Leshner famously published "Addiction Is a Brain Disease, and It Matters."[2] In it, he argued that "dramatic advances over the past two decades in both the neurosciences and behavioral sciences have revolutionized our understanding of drug abuse and addiction. . . . Research has also begun to reveal major differences between the brains of addicted and non-addicted individuals and to indicate some common elements of addiction, regardless of the substance."[3]

At the time, Leshner directed the National Institute on Drug Abuse (NIDA), which funded more than 85 percent of the world's research on addiction and drug abuse.[4] As noted, this view of addiction secured great increases in funding for its research.

Surgeon General Vivek Murthy, in a 2016 essay in the *New England Journal of Medicine*, declares the Neuroscience model of addiction to be a fact: "And perhaps most important, we can use our position as leaders in society to change how society sees addiction—not as a personal failure but as a *chronic disease of the brain* that requires compassion and care" (emphasis added).[5]

The preceding chapter explained how some of the major claims of AA and NA's famous model of alcoholism and addiction may be false. This chapter does similar work with the Neuroscience model, which has captured the most funding and attention of scientists over the past decades, but which also has significant problems.

ESSENTIAL CLAIMS OF THE NEUROSCIENCE MODEL

Like Alcoholics/Narcotics Anonymous, the Neuroscience model contains specific claims about addiction. Volkow and Leshner make at least three separate claims: (1) that addiction is a disease, like other diseases treated by physicians, (2) that addiction is a disease not of the liver or kidneys, but rather a disease of the brain, and (3) that it is an *acquired* disease of the brain. As we shall see, other neuroscience researches also claim that (4) addiction and alcoholism *permanently* damage the brain.

As Neil Levy notes, the Neuroscience model makes not only factual but also moral claims.[6] For example, Leshner laments the stigma attached to addiction and the view that "addicts are weak or bad people, unwilling to lead moral lives and to control their behavior and gratifications." Volkow agrees: "The concept of addiction as a disease of the brain challenges deeply ingrained values about self-determination and personal responsibility that frame drug use as a voluntary, hedonistic act."[7] Neurobiologists want both the solid factual ground of best knowledge of science and the high moral ground of most compassionate view of addiction.

The philosopher Ludwig Wittgenstein once wrote, "Beware the first steps in an ongoing philosophical debate," by which he meant to beware the frame in which your opponent constructs the debate because it may trap you in incorrect assumptions.

Two facts that lie in dispute here are whether addiction is *always* and *only* a disease of the brain. Researchers in neuroscience defend this view passionately and without qualification. In his 2018 text, *The Science of Addiction: From Neurobiology to Treatment*, neuroscientist Carlton Erickson writes, "Excellent scientific research in . . . the past 25 years clearly shows that addiction is a chronic, medical brain disease."[8]

By imaging the flow of blood in the brain of heavy cocaine users, researchers claimed that these users suffered reduced flow of blood to their prefrontal cortex, a problem that lasted as long as ten days after users stopped taking cocaine.[9] From such studies, neurobiologists then assert two further claims: that addicts suffer pathological changes in the deep pathways of their brain which (5) create cravings and (6) make it impossible for addicts to give up their drug usage just by willpower.

There is nothing new in the claim that addicts and alcoholics suffer from cravings for their favorite substance and that overcoming cravings is difficult to do. What is exciting, what has grabbed the attention of the media, and what has gotten funding from NIH, are the claims that the *structure of the brain* has been permanently changed. Thus, as Leshner writes, "a major goal in treatment must be either to reverse or compensate for those brain changes."[10] As such, other treatments, focusing on external behavior or willpower, will only be superficial, although some external behaviors may change.

Since Leshner's article, researchers have focused on a *reward pathway* in the brain, the "mesolimbic dopamine system (MDS)," and the release of dopamine. Disruptive changes in the MDS from drugs or alcohol damage neurotransmitters and create impaired control over drug use.[11] More technically, the infusion of drugs such as opiates overloads the brain with dopamine, so the brain itself reduces release of dopamine or reduces the number of dopamine receptors or the neurons produce less dopamine.[12] "Initially, drug use is voluntary . . . but when the switch is thrown, the individual moves into the state of addiction, characterized by compulsive drug seeking and use."[13]

Over the last decades, researchers acquired expensive new tools for imaging blood flow to the brain, such as positron emission tomography (PET) and fMRI (functional Magnetic Resonance Imaging) scanning.[14] From images generated from such imaging tools, and perhaps to secure more funding, researchers made bold claims about alcoholism and addiction.

Of course, ordinary people don't know how to evaluate such claims, but here's a heads-up about what is to come: let's not be intimidated by technical language about the brain or by colored lights on scans associated with blood flow in the brain.

Here is a typical example of a claim by neurosciences about addiction: A study publicized in 2019 claimed that a single dose of cocaine alters the perineuronal net (PNN), which covers some neurons associated with addiction. "It doesn't take much cocaine to alter the circuit," said Sue Aicher, PhD, a professor of physiology and pharmacology of the School of Medicine at the Oregon Health Sciences University.[15] Because these nets are found in areas of the brain associated with attention, memory, and learning, damage to these nets from a single dose of cocaine are claimed to have important implications for susceptibility to addiction. And, of course, repeated use of cocaine would be expected to increase the damage. This example implies that addiction *permanently* changes in the brain.

Neurobiologists usually make several more specific claims about how addiction comes about in the brain. First, there is the early, potent release of dopamine in the ecstasy of the first-time high. For some users, especially ones who may have suffered lifelong depression or long bouts of chronic pain, this first-time high may be the first time they felt truly at peace.

Unfortunately for users, continued drug usage results in "down regulation" of receptors of dopamine—that is, they disappear or integrate, becoming fewer, such that from the same amount of dopamine, addicts over months or years at some point no longer experience euphoria. But then, according to neurobiologists, a second, biological process has been embedded: "In the addicted brain, the anti-reward system becomes overactive, giving rise to the highly dysphoric phase of drug addiction that ensues when the direct effects of the drug wear off or the drug is withdrawn."[16]

Exactly what it means to say "the anti-reward system becomes overactive" may seem vague, but the phrase implies that the structure of the brain has changed. This change explains a paradox in the behavioral cycle of addiction and alcoholism—namely, that users continue to use these drugs even though it no longer brings them any pleasure to do so. And why do they do so? The answer is not that they still are chasing that first high, but rather that they are now escaping the painful after-effects of using narcotics or alcohol. In other words, now they are using not to get high but to feel normal again.

This is a significant insight and, regardless of what the Neuroscience model says about anything else, it remains an important fact for any therapist treating alcoholism or addiction.

Finally, for neurobiologists, this chasing of the first high and this desire to avoid the pain of withdrawal eventually changes the structure or function of the brain, resulting in damage to higher-level thinking and leading to many poor judgments about family, work, and risk-benefit ratios. And if the first high occurs in adolescence, when thrill seeking and immaturity rule, addiction may result. (Some studies suggest that giving narcotics after removal of wisdom teeth may lead teenagers into addiction, who may think, "This is how I was meant to feel."[17])

THE NEUROSCIENCE OF FREE WILL

Neuroscience seems to have no room for free will. The neuroscience of free will is a hot topic in philosophy and neuroscience. Philosopher Gregg Caruso argues that recent empirical studies in neuroscience, cognitive science, and behaviorism support the conclusion that free will is an "illusion."[18]

Benjamin Libet's disturbing studies in 1983 seemed to show that a brain potential related to movement occurred *before* participants reported being aware of their conscious intention to move. As a result, some neuroscientists doubted whether conscious decisions actually caused a person to move his limbs or body.[19] Some neuroscientists claim that the conscious feeling of making decisions is merely *epiphenomenal*, the idea that, despite our intuitions to the contrary, conscious decisions are powerless over bodily mechanisms, not real, causally efficacious powers, merely the superficial manifestations of underlying brain activity.

For example, biochemical changes in the gut signal that more energy (food) is required, sending signals up the brain that then manifest in an agent's conscious mind: "I should get something to eat now." Others feeling stress may experience the thought "I'm going for a run now to feel better." Of course, for those who experimented with alcohol or opiates, the thoughts may be more urgent: "I must get a drink or some stuff NOW!"

In the decades since 1983, philosophers and neuroscientists have sparred over interpreting Libet's experiments and its subsequent replications. They disagree about the meaning of his research and about what conclusions can be drawn from them about free will. This sparring mirrors the previous question about how much can be inferred about brain function from brain scans.

Let's take a larger view here for a moment. Fifty years ago, the behavioral explanations of addiction ruled, especially in terms of classical and operational conditioning. Also figuring heavily in explanations of alcoholism in medical sociology were descriptions of social roles involving drug users, drug pushers, and deviant behavior. Following that, we witnessed an era in which environmental causes were emphasized, especially as causes of diseases, including alcoholism and addiction.

In the twenty-first century, the pendulum swung to the opposite pole when scientists ditched external explanations for internal ones. The "decade of the brain" began, followed by a new focus on evolutionary explanations and genetics. This switch seemed to mirror Kuhn's famous idea in *The Structure of Scientific Revolutions* that science periodically undergoes major paradigm shifts.

Recently, however, Libet's studies have come under attack for *presupposing* a view antithetical to free will rather than *proving* a lack of free will.[20] In a sustained review of such studies, experts in neuroethics concluded, "We found that interpretation of study results appears to have been driven by the metaphysical position the given author or authors subscribed to—not by a careful analysis of the results themselves. Basically, those who opposed free will interpreted the results to support their position, and vice versa."[21]

Notice that, again, the problem here is the validity of an inference from either external behavior or a certain technical marker of brain activity to what is really going on internally with thinking, consciousness, and free will.

Finally, one more major problem remains with any claim in neuroscience that free will does not exist, and it is on the practical level. If we are trying to help heavy drinkers and addicted people recover, and we claim that they lack free will, what is the point of therapy or urging people to change? Despite our views about the falsity of free will, do we adopt a "strategic stance" in counseling that addicted people really have free will? That seems to take away the moral high ground in applying neuroscience to addiction medicine. It may also be an insurmountable problem for those in addiction medicine, for counselors, and for family members of substance abusers.

AN EVOLUTIONARY BASIS OF ADDICTION?

One might think that the destructive aspects of addiction would not be reinforced in human evolution, but at least one professor of neuroscience argues the opposite. Judy Grisel, a recovering addict, behavioral neuroscientist, and professor of psychology at Bucknell University in Lewisburg, argues in her essay in *Scientific American* (and her book) that addiction often begins with thrill seeking by bored people.[22] Combined with substantial numbers of their opposites, thrill-avoiding people, our thrill-seeking ancestors tried new things, and by doing so, sometimes gave their progeny evolutionary advantages:

> A core attribute of addictive drugs is that they are neurologically newsworthy, and for sensation-seekers, they may satisfy a craving like scratching an itch. Though a tendency to spend the rent money on a transient solution to boredom might be hard to fathom as a parent or partner of such an individual, from an evolutionary perspective, such tendencies may be a real asset.[23]

Here we have a larger claim than just that repeated use of opioids alters the user's brain. Here we have a claim deeper than the inside/outside the body claim discussed before. Here we have the claim that a certain type of personality, one prone to thrill seeking (and hence, a greater risk of addiction), is deep-wired in our genes through the billions of reproductive acts that stand behind human evolution. Grisel: "This means that addiction is a consequence of the biologically driven states inherent in a great many of us."[24]

Other neuroscientists have made similar, speculative claims.[25] One was from Ronald Siegel, a professor of psychiatry and behavioral sciences at UCLA who studied psychoactive substances and who believed that the desire to get high "was permanently and deeply embedded in the psyche of every human being."[26] Siegel claimed that "the war on drugs is a war against ourselves, a denial of our very nature."[27] He claimed that in addition to the three primal drives of sex, hunger, and thirst, the desire to get high was a "fourth drive," inherent to all humans and most animals.

How far will this go? Patricia Churchland, a philosopher, claims morality is based in neurobiology because moral activities, such as caring for children and cooperation at staff meetings, cause pleasurable brain chemicals, such as oxytocin and dopamine, to be released.[28] Certainly Kant, as well as anyone raising bratty children or who's attended a raucous faculty meeting, would be amused.

CRITICISMS OF NEUROSCIENCE

Let's start with Grisel's claim that addiction may have evolved because risk-taking genes offer some evolutionary advantage. What are we to make of such a claim? Is it scientific, or just using scientific ideas to speculate? (Could addicts excuse themselves by saying, "My ancestors made me do it"?)

However, from an evolutionary perspective, why couldn't the opposite be argued with equal persuasion? Why not argue that those with thrill-seeking genes took too many chances as adolescents and died before they could secure mates to pass on their genes? Those with thrill-avoiding genes stayed home, found mates, and passed on their genes many times over, securing a future for thrill-avoiding genes in countless progeny.

Some scientists accuse philosophers of useless speculation, but if we can easily argue the role of thrill-seeking genes in opposite ways in evolution, with no controlled studies available for evidence either way, what is the point of the claim? Professor Grisel postulates a mix of thrill-seeking ancestors with their opposites. Such a mix makes it hard, even impossible, to imagine what might count as evidence for or against this claim, and that is a bad thing for an allegedly scientific hypothesis.

DEEPER PROBLEMS WITH THE NEUROSCIENCE MODEL

Now let's consider other problems in the Neuroscience model. As hinted, a crucial one concerns exactly what can, and cannot, be inferred from new images of blood flow in the brain. Consider the following claim in *Overcoming Opioid Addiction* (2018), by Adam Bisaga, a physician who specializes in addiction psychiatry at Columbia University:

> But the evidence does not lie. Brain-imaging studies that evaluated areas of the brain involved in maintaining uncontrollable drug use show changes in function as compared to otherwise healthy brains, just as imaging studies show decreased function in the areas of heart muscle where blood flow is blocked. In parallel, studies show reversal of these "abnormal" changes in the brains of patients who are able to remain drug free for more than six months as compared with the brains of patients with only days of abstinence. . . . The fact that there is a predictable brain activity with the emergence and resolution of the disorder supports the fact that at the core of addiction is a disordered brain.[29]

Does the analogy between decreased blood flow to the heart and decreased blood flow to an area of the brain hold? Obviously, the areas of the brain are not *permanently* damaged, or no addict would ever cease using and recover.

Even this quotation recognizes that addiction can be overcome and that damage (as measured by blood flow) can be reversed.

However, unlike the heart, we know that when one area of the brain is damaged, other areas can take over. Do we know whether this happens with decreased blood flow to one area of the brain?

Some neuroscientists distinguish between damage to the brain's structure versus damage to its function. There may be permanent structural damage from addiction and alcoholism, but some function can be partially (or even fully) recovered.

Next, if there is less flow to a particular region of the brain during and after use of cocaine or heroin, does that necessarily show that this area is damaged? In their review of studies of the neuroscience of addiction, philosophers of science Harold Kincaid and Jacqueline Sullivan agree that the predominant medical model in research revolves around describing the mesolimbic dopamine system, which functions at multiple levels, from molecules to behavior. This model, they assert, is a "bold, interesting and parsimonious hypothesis that is the result of integration of research findings and methodologies across multiple levels of analysis."[30]

In Leshner's seminal article, he claimed, "The common brain effects of addicting substances suggest common brain mechanisms underlying all addictions."[31] But Kincaid and Sullivan question whether his model does what it purports to do: (1) locate with evidence addiction in specific, damaged areas of the brain and (2) explain major aspects of addiction with reference to the same brain neuroadaptations.[32] If the Neuroscience model fails on these two crucial aspects, it has major weaknesses.

Let's deconstruct these claims into the simplest possible language: (1) *craving* is emotional, conscious, internal, and feels like something on which free will must be focused to resist; (2) behavioral compulsions to seek drugs are semiconscious, external, and feel like attacks on free will; (3) damaged neurotransmitters in the MDS system, which supposedly cause addiction, are biological, internal, mechanistic, and presuppose no free will. The important point is that it's a big jump to explaining how (1) and (2) connect to (3).

Along this general skeptical line, consider the critique of neuroscience by Yale psychiatrist Sally Satel and Emory psychologist Scott Lilienfeld:

Now introduce brain imaging, which seems to serve up visual proof that addiction is a brain disease. But neurobiology is not destiny: the disruptions in neural mechanisms associated with addiction do constrain a person's capacity for choice, but they do not destroy it. What's more, training the spotlight too intently on the workings of the addicted brain leaves the addicted person in the shadows, distracting clinicians, policy makers, and sometimes patients themselves from other powerful psychological and environmental forces that exert strong influence on them.[33]

In other words, the Neuroscience model is reductionistic: it makes human decisions and their consequences just the result of neurons firing and their communications with each other. In particular, this model claims that decisions by addicted adults are the result of neurons *damaged* by narcotics or alcohol and their *mis*-communication with each other.

Note that this account of addiction and alcoholism in neuroscience might describe only 1–2 percent of heavy users who feel they are in the grip of something overpowering. There may be adverse selection about what kind of addicted person is studied. As Sally Satel and Scott Lilienfeld note, heavily addicted patients are the ones most often seen by psychiatrists, but they are not representative of all addicted people. So it might be in error to generalize what is true of addicts or heavy drinkers in treatment to all drinkers and drug users.

THE PROBLEM OF SPONTANEOUS REMISSION

Another problem with the Neuroscience model (and every model except Harm Reduction) is almost never discussed among neuroscientists, just as a similar problem is rarely discussed among those who treat alcoholics. As noted in the previous chapter, Fingarette discovered that regardless of which treatment they used, *most heavy drinkers learned to control their drinking*. Even more amazingly, he discovered that "about one third of all heavy drinkers, including those diagnosed as alcoholics, improve over time *without any treatment*" (emphasis added).[34]

Similarly, for those addicted to opioids, Kincaid and Sullivan note that "the rates of *spontaneous remission* among diagnosed addicts are actually quite high."[35] The key phrase here in the literature of addiction is "spontaneous remission," a misleading phrase borrowed from oncology; in this context it refers to allegedly compulsive drug users who stop using without formal treatment.[36] It is damaging enough for neuroscience that addicted people can stop using without replacement medications, but it is even worse that they can stop *without being in any rehabilitation program at all*. In contrast, if you have the disease of cardiomyopathy, your heart does not suddenly get better, especially without drugs or rehabilitation.

How can the Neuroscience model possibly explain such a high rate of remissions? How can it explain *any* spontaneous remissions at all? If the brain has been permanently damaged by a pattern of release of dopamine along the mesolimbic pathway, how can it suddenly recover?

Obviously, neuroscience cannot maintain the claim that addiction irrevocably alters the brain. It's just not factual. The history of the problem goes back to what Sally Satel and Scott Lilienfeld call the dogma "promoted tirelessly by psychologist Alan I. Leshner, then the director of the National Institute on Drug Abuse," that "once an addict, always an addict."[37]

One way out for neuroscientists is to claim that, yes, the brain's structure has been altered by addiction or alcoholism, but because the brain has plasticity, alternative neural pathways can be activated in partial or full recovery. This allegedly explains how many people in their mid-thirties learn to control their drinking or injections.

But this explanation seems very ad hoc. Because we know that lots of people recover on their own, neuroscientists claim that they must have developed alternative neural pathways (or functions) to enable them to cope without drugs or alcohol. But how do we know that? Is it just a guess? What would falsify the claim? Or is it non-falsifiable?

The depth of this problem cannot be overemphasized. In medical-biological models of addiction or alcoholism, it should be very difficult for people just to stop drinking or just to stop injecting. If addiction is truly a disease of the brain, whether it affects structure or primordial functions, no one should be able to experience an existential crisis and quit. And yet this happens (among others, see the example in chapter 8 of Sherman Alexie's mother).

In an essay in the *New York Times*, two famous journalists, noted addiction journalist Maia Szalawitz and addiction photographer Ryan Christopher Jones, emphasized how most people with addictions recover, often on their own:

A large national population study found that almost all of those who once met the criteria for prescription opioid-use disorder achieved remission during their lifetimes—and half of those recovered within five years. Although heroin and fentanyl are more dangerous than prescription opioids, most of those who avoid fatal overdoses recover from addiction.[38]

Why do we so rarely hear these facts? Regardless of whether these people quit on their own or after various therapies, the problem remains of explaining how reversal of supposedly permanent damage occurs.

Spontaneous remission famously occurred when veterans returned from the Vietnam War. In Asia, some soldiers used heroin; alarmists predicted that when they returned, they would still be addicted to heroin, but this was true only for a small minority. Back in the States, most simply stopped using, without any formal program.

Interestingly, although neuroscience rarely discusses this result, the field itself provides a possible explanation for spontaneous remission (a.k.a. "maturing out"). It is a well-known fact that the adolescent brain differs substantially from an adult's thirty-five-year-old brain. For example, researchers Mariam Arain et al. write in 2013 in *Neuropsychiatric Disease and Treatment*:

> The maturation of the adolescent brain is also influenced by heredity, environment, and sex hormones (estrogen, progesterone, and testosterone), which play a crucial role in myelination. Furthermore, glutamatergic neurotransmission predominates, whereas gamma-aminobutyric acid neurotransmission remains under construction, and this might be responsible for immature and impulsive behavior and neurobehavioral excitement during adolescent life. . . . Prenatal neglect, cigarette smoking, and alcohol consumption may also significantly impact maturation of the adolescent brain.[39]

It is well known that most abusers of alcohol and opiates begin young and that most middle-age adults learn to control the extremes of drinking and drug usage. Whether one interprets this physically (in terms of incomplete myelination of the brain) or mentally (the person's character grows), the most obvious explanation for spontaneous remission among heavy users of alcohol and opiates is that adults around age thirty-five find themselves making important decisions about whether to throw their lives away on drugs or alcohol or begin to live a normal, adult life.

THE LIMITS OF EXPLANATION IN NEUROSCIENCE

Several prominent psychologists, such as György Buzsáki, reject the trend in neuroscience to label scans of blood flow in the brain with mental states in humans. As the distinguished psychologist, Jerome Kagan, wrote in 2017:

> Brain states consist of continually changing patterns of voltages, frequencies, and molecular deformations of varying numbers of neurons at distinctive locations of

varying durations. Although these states are the foundation of all psychological phenomena, it is impossible at the moment to explain how the latter emerge from the former.[40]

Kagan harshly criticizes the trend in neuroscience of applying familiar terms for conscious human states—such as aggression, fear, shyness, top-down control, or craving—to brain states: "The practice of borrowing concepts with distinctive meaning and validities when they refer to human psychological processes and applying them to animals or brains is reminiscent of the labels of early-nineteenth century phrenologists gave to locations on the skull."[41]

Dualism is not fashionable these days in neuroscience, psychology, or even parts of philosophy, but we feel a difference between what happens in our brains when we feel hungry and the conscious decision "I am going to eat now." Similarly, Kagan writes, "the term *fear* presupposes a conscious human agent and should not be used to describe a brain profile." Moreover, "the meaning of the predicate *fears* in a sentence describing the emotion of a woman who avoids parties differs from the meaning of the same word in a sentence describing the increased BOLD signal to the amygdala of an adult looking at pictures of snakes and spiders" lying still and supine in the narrow tube of an MRI scanner.[42]

This is not a new problem. Scientists studying the brain have always tended to be materialists, seeking a physical lesion or pathway for each mental event. Although this methodology worked well with schizophrenia, it has not always done so. The foundational idea of Sigmund Freud, that some patients could improve by talking about past trauma or abuse (his so-called "talking cure"), was rejected for years by most physicians of his time, who sought anatomical causes for psychiatric disorders.[43]

Another case in point may be the very idea of a mature brain. Maturity is a concept predicated on a scale of observable human actions, from extreme risk taking for silly goals to taking calculated risks for courageous goals. Although it is appropriate to describe a brain as larger, having more volume, having more neurons, or being more active, it is unclear what it means to say a brain developed in such-and-such a way *causes* mature behavior.[44] Do mature brains process dopamine faster or slower than immature brains? Do the brains of some people get stuck and not mature? Is an immature brain the cause or result of using opiates heavily in adolescence?

All in all, although we clearly know what it means to say that an adolescent has put aside his foolish way, it is unclear whether "a mature brain" has any clear *biological*, *anatomical*, or *physiological* meaning.

CRITICISMS OF THE NEUROSCIENCE MODEL
FROM OTHER MODELS

The success of the Neuroscience model in getting funding, the audacity of some of its claims, and the lack of its practical applicability in ordinary therapy mean that many champions of opposing models believe it needs to be taken down a peg, not just for its orientation but also for the way its champions comport themselves and their failure to include other views as worthy of respect.

From the perspective of the Coping model (to be discussed later), the Neuroscience model has another problem—namely, devaluing the social context in which addiction and heavy drinking occurs. (To be fair, Leshner admits that the social context of addiction matters a lot, citing the Vietnam veterans who only used in Vietnam.) Coping model counselors argue that when neuroscientists claim that drug dealers get a dopamine rush when they unload a new batch of drugs or that thrill seeking by addicts creates a need for rushes of dopamine, it is at best half the story. What is needed is an appreciation for how alcoholism and addiction develop in specific contexts and how, in other contexts, it can be overcome or moderated.

CONCLUSIONS

Given the Neuroscience model's lack of answers to the problem of spontaneous remission, it fails major requirements of a good model of addiction: (1) it doesn't prove the connections between images of decreased blood flow and damage to the brain; (2) it doesn't prove connections between that alleged damage to the brain and craving for drugs; (3) it doesn't explain how or why many substance abusers learn to control their usage or quit; (4) it ignores the personal and social factors in using alcohol and opiates.

In addition, the claims of some researches that long-term drinking and opiate usage permanently alters the brain appears to be false, at least if "permanently alters" means that such drinking and usage can never stop.

Summary of the Neuroscience Model

Underlying cause: The alcoholic and addict both suffer from a disease just as real as renal failure or cardiac myopathy. Both heavy drinking and use of narcotics over the years changes the structure of the brain. Because of such deep, structural change, those affected find it impossible to escape their destructive behavior. Because those affected are experiencing altered brain states, they cannot make rational decisions about risk and reward, impairing their relationships with others.

Treatment: Target the underlying changes in the brain and attempt to reverse that damage. Research by neurologists, psychiatrists, and neurobiologists should focus on understanding and reversing these structural changes. Of the utmost importance to the Neuroscience model is that no treatment is realistic that does not help the patient reduce cravings. From a pharmacological view of the pathology of the brain, the only effective way to so reduce craving is to prescribe drugs such as benzodiazepines that mute the intensity of the cravings.

Other models: They make a major mistake in not treating the underlying biochemical changes in the brain. For neuroscientists, AA/NA errs in thinking that religious conversion, fellowship, buddies, and willpower are enough to overcome alcoholism and addiction. For most people, they are not. Although these may help some victims, without reducing the biological craving, success will not come.

Responsibility: Alcoholics and addicts are victims who are not responsible for contracting their diseases, just as those afflicted by brain cancer are not responsible for their sickness. Even if choice was involved in the past (for example, in smokers who get various kinds of cancer), physicians should not give such patients moralistic sermons.

Family matters: Obviously, if alcoholism and addiction are diseases of the brain, where deep structures inside the brain have changed, the important thing to do is to prevent such changes and try to reverse them. What goes on outside the brain, or outside the substance abuser, is tangential.

POOR CHOICES

> Here was the secret of happiness, about which philosophers had disputed for so many ages, at once discovered; happiness might now be bought for a penny and carried in the waistcoat-pocket; portable ecstasies might be had corked up in a pint-bottle; and peace of mind could be sent down by the mail.
>
> —Thomas De Quincey, *Confessions of an English Opium-Eater* (1821)

I will call the model "Kantian" to have a useful way of referring to an approach that emphasizes the power of persons to make changes. I could also call it "Buddhist model," "Insight model," "Rational Recovery model," or "Mindfulness-Based Relapse Prevention model."[1] Similarly, the addictive voice recognition technique, which resembles meditation exercises in yoga and Buddhism used to tame the "beast" of addictive craving, falls under this model. When it comes to stopping drinking or using drugs, all these models agree that the major problem is not only physical but also *mental*.

All these models reject epiphenomenalism. All believe in the power of minds over hidden forces—forces such as behavioral conditioning, neurosynaptic activity, or biochemical processes. Where neuroscience might focus on neurological repair, Kantians focus on mental refocusing.

IMMANUEL KANT

Although Kant did not write much about addiction or alcoholism, he did mention these topics. I believe the label "Kantian" for this model is appropriate.

Immanuel Kant (1724–1804) lived almost three hundred years ago in Konigsberg, Prussia (now Germany). He lived during the Enlightenment, a time when people believed in reason and what it could achieve. His ideas on individual autonomy and reason helped fuel later political revolutions in France and America.

Raised by pious, Christian parents, Kant at university felt conflict between the biblical and scientific accounts of Creation. He originally studied topology but switched to philosophy to discover whether religious belief could be made compatible with science. His *Critique of Pure Reason* (1781) laid out his conclusions, where he critiqued the limits of reason "to make room for faith."

In his *Metaphysics of Morals*, Kant has a section titled "On Stupefying One-self by the Excessive Use of Food or Drink," in which he writes:

> A human being who is drunk is like a mere animal, not to be treated as a human being. . . . It is obvious that putting oneself in such a state violates a duty to oneself. The first of these debasements, below even the nature of an animal, is usually brought about by fermented drinks, but it can also result from other narcotics, such as opium, and other vegetable products. They are seductive because, under their influence, people dream for a while that they are happy and free from care, and even imagine that they are strong; but dejection and weakness follow and, worst of all, they create the need to use the narcotics again and even to increase the amount.[2]

Kant found a little wine or beer acceptable, which he thought could "promote sociability and conversation," but in his *Lectures on Ethics* he argued that the body must be trained to control any desire for alcohol or opium: "The body must first be disciplined, because it contains principles which affect the mind and can change its condition. . . . The mind need only secure that the body does not exercise any compulsion upon it."[3]

Kant goes on to stress that in such discipline of the body, "the body must be made frugal in its needs and temperate in its pleasures." Moreover, "the vices of over-eating and over-drinking are bestial and degrade man." Social drinking is permissible for Kant, but "secret drinking, drunkenness in solitude, is as disgraceful [as gluttony], for then the factor [of sociability] which raised it a fraction above gluttony disappears." For Kant, virtue is about control of the mind over the habits of the body.

KANT'S VIEW OF THE PERSON

Kant articulated an ethical model that continues to be important today. It gives robust moral standing to persons. One of his most famous statements, which goes to the heart of his view, is "Act so that you treat humanity, whether in your own person or in that of another, always as an end and never as a means only."[4]

When Kant urged us to treat people always as an end and never as a means, he is asserting that humans have intrinsic value, not derivative or extrinsic value. Kant recognized the duality of human nature, the fact that humans combine both a physical nature governed by laws of natural sciences, and a mental nature, where a deep self or soul hosts the seat of rationality, free will, spirituality, and morality.

As a thing, a human body can be thought of scientifically: As a biological organism, human bodies are subject to the laws of evolution and mitosis; as a chemical entity, human bodies can be analyzed as chemicals in motion; and as an object of physics, they can be seen like something thrown out a window, things that obey the laws of gravity in falling to the ground. But as non-physical *persons*, humans for Kant are much grander than animals and possess inherent dignity.

It is important to understand not only *what* Kant thought about the value of humans but also *why*. Humans are special because of their unique qualities. First, they are *rational*, meaning they are capable of weighing reasons, evaluating evidence, and reflecting on the best path to a goal. Second, they possess *free will*, meaning they can rise above their animal nature, their psychological conditioning, and social roles to make genuinely free decisions. Third, they are capable of rising above self-interest and doing the right thing simply because moral duty requires it. That is, they are capable of being *true moral agents*. Finally, they possess a deep self (some call it a soul) that is the subject of consciousness, conscience, reflection, and free will, making humans unique in the animal kingdom. For all these reasons, humans have moral value, unique in the world we know.

All of these distinctively human qualities ground the crucial importance of autonomy in Kantian ethics. In the context of drinking and addiction, Kant believes humans can be "law-givers unto themselves" or, alternatively, give up on themselves, treating themselves as mere objects. But in doing the latter, they destroy something that is part of their essence.

It does not matter to Kant if most humans abuse their natures and if most do not act according to their highest nature. Even if most people act irrationally, selfishly, and as though they had no free will, Kant prefers to base his model on what humans *can* achieve and how they *can* act, not on how they *actually act*.

Because each human is special, all humans are special. From this simple truth, enormous ethical obligations ensue. Each of us has a strict obligation to treat other humans as fully autonomous, as equal moral agents, to not harm other humans, to go to the aid of injured humans, and, in all ways, to respect humanity and persons therein.

For Kant, the most important flaw of the disease model of alcoholism/ addiction would be its treatment of persons as mere things. That is, it treats a heavy drinker as the cumulative result of the causal forces acting on her body and personality, such that her drinking inevitably flows from these causes. For Kant, this account loses the essence of persons—their rationality, their conscious reflection, and their real choices each day in bringing alcohol to their lips.

Although this may sound harsh, Kant thinks that holding a person responsible for his actions is the only way to treat him with respect. Kant famously held that the only way to treat a murderer with respect was by capital punishment. Even if the world is about to end, the murderer must still be punished, not as a mean to deter others but to give him what he deserves. For these reasons, Kantians will hold the addicted person and heavy drinker responsible for his actions in ways that biological models will not.

Some modern programs for treating alcoholism and addiction are Kantian in emphasizing mindfulness or refocusing thoughts. These methods agree with Kant and emphasize that mental control is within most people's grasp. For example, Darren Littlejohn, a recovering addict who became a psychologist and Zen practitioner, grafts Tibetan Buddhism onto twelve-step programs to help people like him gain control of cravings, using meditation to create calmness, and overall, using meditation to overcome the intense mental obsessions of the addicted mind.[5] Likewise, psychiatrist Judson Brewer combines Buddhist techniques with psychiatry in his mindfulness-based relapse prevention (MBRP) program.[6]

Exactly how mental control is gained in the above programs is not important for Kant. For Kant, each is just tweaking mental powers, and it's likely that different techniques will work for different people. Whether we call these techniques "Buddhist," "rational-emotive therapy," "Christian feedback," or "self-insight exercises," the point is to gain mental control over obsessive thoughts.

Kant would applaud all these programs because they all oppose the disease model assumed by the AA/NA, Neuroscience, and Genetics models. In these models, substance abusers are victims, on whom bigger forces operate to cause them to harm themselves, not agents who could make better choices.

And here is precisely the second problem for Kantians. People *do* have free will, and to treat them as if they do not is to treat them badly, to treat them like animals or things, and such treatment demeans their humanity. Sure, they chose to drink, or to inject heroin, and sure, they become dependent on these substances, but that doesn't mean they have forever lost their ability to choose otherwise. All of us make choices every day, including the choice to buy another bottle of whiskey or to meet the drug pusher for the next hit.

Indeed, for Kant, Alcoholics Anonymous and neuroscience contradict themselves because their recovery programs assume that each victim has the power to choose to recover. When AA or NA agrees with Kant and holds users responsible for their past actions and makes them apologize to their victims, aren't the users assuming personal responsibility for past actions and implying that they could have acted differently? If the disease controlled everything, what's the point of making amends to family and friends hurt by your bad past behavior?

When people claim it's a virtue that scientific models remove stigma from users and see them as victims, not as moral failures, Kant demurs. What exactly does it mean to "remove stigma"? Is it to hold someone blameless who secretly took out a $200,000 loan and spent all the money on heroin, leaving his spouse and children homeless? Can the spouse not justifiably ask, "How could you do this to us?"

For Kantians, it's also hard to make AA's view of alcoholism consistent: If you're by nature sinful or weak, and therefore succumbed to the disease, how can you overcome it? Regardless of theological beliefs, one can respect the power within us. If AA claims that you can overcome addiction only by calling on a Higher Power, why can't you call on that same power by yourself without AA?

Which raises the thorny question: Exactly what is it to say that such-and-such a condition is a "disease"? Certainly, that word in medicine has major connotations, implying that physicians should treat the condition, that victims should be treated by physicians in hospitals or special clinics, and, importantly, that health insurance should reimburse physicians for treating this condition.

The way AA thinks of alcoholism/addiction as a disease posits a radically different kind of disease than, say, cystic fibrosis, where free will plays no role in contracting it. Perhaps a kinder view of AA/NA is to say that they assume that free will is a necessary but not a sufficient condition for kicking alcohol or narcotics.

Finally, the Kantian model emphasizes that the right thing to do is universalizable. That is, we should generalize the rule we are acting on so that all of humanity can and should act on the same rule. If we treat alcoholics as people who are not responsible for their actions because they have a disease, then what else should we absolve all of humanity of because their actions may also have prior causes?

Put differently, disease models of alcoholism cannot be the real solution to curing alcoholism, *but for Kant, it is itself part of the real problem.* It is part of the problem because it ignores the key fact that must be accepted for an alcoholic to change: that he or she must consciously *decide* to change and to *decide* each day to stay sober.[7]

For Kantians, the Neuroscience model suffers the same problem because it downplays, or even ignores, the central role of the agent in change. The more Neuroscience paints addiction like schizophrenia, the more both agents and their families see a loss of control, but such a loss is false to the actual life trajectory of most users.

Also, ignoring the centrality of free will in human lives and in morality explains the growing tendency to see everyone as a victim. Kant would despise this cultural phenomenon of seeing everyone as addicted to something, because these trends undermine human dignity and freedom. In a real sense, if you make a person think he is a victim, he feels like one. However, if you make the person think he is responsible for himself, he will feel that way, too. Kant's insight is the moral truth behind many youth programs that try to teach personal responsibility and having pride in exercising control over their own lives and bodies.

THE BUDDHIST VERSION OF KANTIAN MODEL

It has not escaped the notice of practitioners of Buddhism both that the mental control needed by heavy drinkers and drug abuser can be obtained through insights taken from this way of life and that some key ideas of Buddhism apply especially to addiction. The most ancient form of this worldview, Theravada Buddhism, stems from the Pāli Canon and emphasizes the Four Noble Truths: (1) life is filled with suffering, (2) suffering is caused by craving for pleasurable sensations and fulfillment of desires, (3) suffering can cease, and (4) the way suffering can cease is the discipline of the eightfold path.

This form of Buddhism is not so much a religion in the Western sense of religion as an anti-religious psychology.[8] Of great importance to alcoholism and addiction is the connection between craving and substance abuse. There are many forms of craving, Siddhartha emphasizes: for sexual conquest, for power, for fame, for food, for social esteem, for long life, for family happiness, and so on. One formula for success is to reduce suffering by reducing cravings, so Buddhist monks in Southeast Asia dress in simple orange robes and beg for food, eschewing power suits and banquets.

Obviously, if techniques are successful for reducing one's list of desires in life, one lessens the chances of being miserable from having unfulfilled desires. Hyper-consumerism and the obsession with social media of modern people would be seen by Siddhartha as yokes to misery. So, too, modern expectations for the perfect career, the blissful marriage, wonderful children who marry the right partner—all of these are portents of great suffering.

In this worldview, craving the pleasures of opiates or alcohol is just one special case of craving and the suffering that comes from not being able to satisfy this special craving is just a subset of the more general kind of suffering. What is always causing suffering is "wanting more," and until that existential desire is extinguished, misery will always follow.

Exactly how all craving is extinguished is a complicated story and one that need not be told here. What is important here is that both Kant and Siddhartha hold that a person has the inner ability to overcome the physical bonds created by craving, and both assert that half the battle of overcoming addiction is just as much mental as it is physical.

LIBERTARIANS, KANT, AND ADDICTION

People who respect free will in ethics may align themselves with similar people in political philosophy who emphasize individual liberty against the powers of the State. Objectivists such as Ayn Rand extol individual liberty and hold individuals responsible for their choices. Ditto for the libertarians, who wish to reduce the imposition of state controls on people and to maximize individual freedom.

As such, libertarians can agree with Kant, but they can be quite harsh in judging people who abuse alcohol and drugs. Yes, some people have become addicted to bad things, libertarians argue, but they have no one to blame but themselves. No one kept forcing them to drink alcohol; no one forced them to try heroin or opiates. And if they end up in bad places, well, that's what happens when people spend a decade making bad choices. Bring in the young people and let them observe what happens when such a decade of bad choices occurs.

Libertarians can also be quite harsh on biological models that excuse drug users and heavy drinkers from personal responsibility. Consider libertarians Satel and Lilienfeld on the Neuroscience model:

> The notion that addiction is a "brain disease" has become widespread and rarely challenged. The brain-disease model implies erroneously that the brain is necessarily the most important and useful level of analysis for understanding and treating addiction. . . . The brain-disease model obscures the dimension of choice in addiction, the capacity to respond to incentives, and also the essential fact people use drugs for reasons (as consistent with a self-medication hypothesis). The latter becomes obvious when patients become abstinent yet still struggle to assume rewarding lives in the realm of work and relationships. Thankfully, addicts can choose to recover and are not helpless victims of their own "hijacked brains."[9]

STRATEGIC VALUE AND FREE WILL

Interestingly, some counselors agree with Kant's emphasis, even while they officially claim alcoholism and addiction as diseases. They talk about *the strategic value* of telling clients they have real choices not to drink and to get better, even if it's not really true. In other words, treat addicts "as if" they have responsibility for their actions, even if you don't believe it or it's false. This is exactly how one scholar concluded his overview of addiction:

> There is an important, but restricted, sense in which the addicted individuals in question are not "responsible" for their decisions regarding drug use. The high likelihood of relapse means that, as a matter of clinical fact, they are usually not accountable. At the same time, clinical experience also suggests that we should treat addicted individuals *as if* they are responsible because that empowerment is often crucial to their recovery.[10]

If it's crucial to their recovery, then doesn't urging free will and the power to change assume that the individuals have the power to recover by being, and feeling, responsible? Is this just a ploy or is it actually a fact? Notice, too, the strange assumption in the above quotation that if a person ever relapses, that person is automatically "not accountable."

The appealing virtue of the Kantian model is that it gives great power to will and the mind. Many recovered alcoholics and addicts write in their memoirs about how the mental struggle to quit was far worse than the physical struggle. People *know* they are destroying their lives, their marriages, their careers. They don't want these things to happen. A mental struggle is constantly occurring. Kant respects that struggle and thinks the mind can win.

As Sally Satel and Scott Lilienfeld write, "The neurocentric view of the mind risks undermining our most deeply held ideas about selfhood, free will, and personal responsibility, putting us at risk of making harmful mistakes, whether in the courtroom, interrogation room, or addiction treatment clinic."[11]

Another advantage of the Kantian model is that, not surprisingly, it thinks that belief in free will is crucial in treating alcoholism and addiction. For Kantians, it matters *a lot* when neuroscientists deny free will. Kant argues that assuming free will is foundational for criminal punishment, raising children, and personal relationships. Where neuroscience espouses what philosopher Gregg Caruso calls "the dark side of free will," Kant espouses the "bright side" that we are truly free.

CRITICISMS OF KANTIAN MODEL BY OTHER MODELS

Any defense of Kant's view among AA counselors usually invokes strong responses. They see the AA way as the only way to stop drinking and view these other models as enabling weak people to continue drinking. What may be closest to the truth is that AA's way works well for a minority of heavy drinkers and its cold-turkey, total-conversion model may be the only model that can help them. Having had such a method work, it is difficult for AA members to believe that Kant could have any part of the truth about drinking or that other methods might work for other drinkers.

From the viewpoint of neuroscience, Kant's view is hopelessly out of date. Where Kant exalts personal autonomy, free will, and the absolute value of the individual, neurobiologists see victims ravaged by a savage disease of the brain. Alcoholics and Narcotics Anonymous agree that victims are afflicted by a disease but disagree about how to treat that disease. For both groups, users must hit bottom, call on a Higher Power to help them quit, stop using, join a group of former users, and engage in the twelve steps to recovery. Substitute medication is not necessary for this journey; indeed, AA/NA discourages substitution of one high for another and points to how cocaine was once seen as a cure for heroin addiction. Maintenance on methadone for AA and NA is not cure but drug switching.

For the Coping model, therapy must address the triggers that cause the addict to seek and use narcotics. It must also break through patterns of denial and self-deception. Ultimately, the user must learn to cope with stress and a life without alcohol and drugs. If such new patterns aren't learned and practiced, drug substitution won't work. What happens in AA/NA groups, according to Coping model, is partly learning how to live without alcohol and drugs.

Geneticists also think Kant's view is outdated. How does Kant explain how alcoholism and addiction run in generations of families? Or how they occur more in certain ethnic groups than others? Advocates of the Social Justice model think Kant's view errs in focusing on individuals and making addiction a moral failing. This view asks, "What is it in that society that helps create so many addicts?" Why do so many alcoholics and addicted people lack meaning in their lives and good jobs? What lack of a safety net lies behind mass addiction?

KANT AND FAMILIES

Parents often blame themselves for the alcoholism or addiction of a child. They are often deeply enmeshed in the life of the child, doing surveillance of the child's activities, paying $40,000 for treatment, and trying to help. As Beverly Conyers writes in *Addict in the Family*, "Often, the harder they try, the more the addict resists their efforts. . . . It is usually much harder for parents . . . to shut the addict out of their lives. Instead, when confronted with addiction, families are often drawn into painful, lengthy, and costly attempts to help the addict get better."[12] And despite all these efforts, Conyers (herself a parent of an addicted daughter) concludes, "Most families are defeated in the end. Addicts persist in their self-destructive, addictive behaviors until *something within themselves*—something quite apart from anyone else's efforts—changes so radically that the desire for a high is dulled and ultimately deadened by a desire for a better life" (emphasis added). Even among those most affected, members of families living with an addicted person or who've lost someone to addiction, only half think addiction is a disease.[13] Kant agrees. No one can force autonomy and free decisions on someone else. Ultimately, the person herself must decide to change.

CONCLUSIONS

In rebuttal to criticisms from other theories, Kantians point to spontaneous remission and how most drinkers and users learn to not descend, as AA claims they must, to rock bottom. These facts seem to partially redeem the Kantian model. Something is going on when a thirty-five-year-old adult "matures out" of his twenty-year affair with binge drinking and becomes a moderate, infrequent drinker. For Kantians, it's the power of the deep self and the acceptance of personal responsibility over one's life.

Virtually every memoir of alcoholism and addiction documents *the mental struggle* to escape dependency. Some drugs, such as cocaine, are physically relatively mild to withdraw from, but forsaking the mental pleasures of cocaine is another story. It is this aspect that Kantians claim is under a person's control.

Are users "bad" who can't control their drinking? Much as it seems at first to be compassionate to adopt ethical relativism or skepticism about such judgments, or to condemn moralism in drug therapy, there is something to be said for not letting those addicted to alcohol or opiates escape retribution for the harm they do to others. The father of Frank McCourt would let his wife and children go without the basic necessities of life, even food, rather than forgo drinking himself to unconsciousness every payday. Is that what a good man does? For Kantians, holding people responsible for the harm they've caused is part of treating them as moral agents and part of the recovery.

Summary of the Kantian Model

Underlying cause: The alcoholic or addict has freely made bad choices and continues to make bad choices each time he uses. He could choose otherwise. When he denies any responsibility for continuing bad behavior, he is in what French philosopher Jean-Paul Sartre called "bad faith." He is treating himself as an object ruled by external causal forces, not as a person endowed with a free, rational soul.

Treatment: No matter whether it is the person herself deciding that the time has come to no longer make drinking or shooting up the central focus of her life, and no matter whether that decision comes after years in therapy with a clinical psychologist or in a group at AA or NA, no change is possible without the affected person owning her past behavior and accepting that she has the power to change. Indeed, Kant insists, *every* model to curing alcoholism and addiction makes this assumption.

Other models: Seeing addiction as a disease or biological fault treats people as objects rather than as free agents who made bad choices. The disease models don't explain how drinkers and users can stop before entering programs or how, once in a program, they can stop. They don't explain why most users stop on their own.

Responsibility: Victims are responsible for their bad choices. It's not just of strategic value in therapy to hold clients responsible for their bad choices, especially choices that destroy relationships and families. It's of the essence of treating others as ends in themselves with inherent dignity to hold them responsible. The dark view of free will is incorrect; people are moral agents who have free will and thus are accountable for their decisions. Because moral responsibility exists and is real, moral blame is also appropriate. Indeed, *not* to blame the alcoholic or addict, *not* to hold them responsible for the damage they do to the lives of their families and friends, and *not* to hold them responsible for the costs of their long-term medical treatment, is to make a grave mistake in moral reasoning and public policy.

Family matters: Relatives can help by holding the substance abuser responsible for his or her actions and not excusing them. They can reject the idea that addiction is a disease and instead see it as a series of continuing bad choices—choices that could be different.

AVOIDING THE WORST OUTCOMES

> Todd was voicing the persistent questions that haunt anyone who has ever loved an addict: "What did I do that caused this problem?" and "What can I do to fix it?" He had not yet discovered the simple truth about addiction that is so hard for families to accept: You didn't cause it, you can't control it, and you can't cure it.
>
> —Beverly Conyers, *Addict in the Family* (2003)

The model of Harm Reduction, a general model in medicine and public health, has much broader applications than just to addiction and alcoholism. A major player in historical fights against syphilis, HIV/AIDS, gambling, prostitution, and infectious diseases, it always clashes with ultraconservative, moralistic models.

This ethical model, like the Neuroscience and part of the AA/NA models, opposes moralistically blaming victims.[1] It thinks we should reduce the bad consequences of deviant behavior rather than try to suppress that behavior. It accepts that people will gamble, hire prostitutes, use dirty needles, and drink too much. It opposes shaming cigarette smokers but advocates encouraging them to use chewing tobacco, nicotine gum, or nicotine patches as less harmful alternatives.

To prevent the spread of syphilis, Harm Reductionists championed giving out condoms during World War I and using penicillin during World War II to cure syphilis. Moralists opposed these approaches, believing that giving out these things would encourage the extramarital sex that caused the spread of syphilis. Harm Reduction can also be employed to reduce harms associated with handguns, teenage pregnancy, smoking, steroids in sports, and malpractice in medicine.[2]

Since the late 1980s, to prevent the spread of HIV/AIDS through the sharing of dirty needles among those who injected drugs, Harm Reductionists championed clean needle-exchange programs. Although strenuously opposed at first by conservative moralists, who argued that such programs encouraged drug usage, by 2019 at least 320 needle exchanges operated in America. They were legal in twenty-eight states and Washington, DC. Such programs now have spread quietly in the forty-eight American counties that account for half of new HIV infections.[3]

Perhaps because of its Puritan heritage and the influence of Alcoholics Anonymous in fighting addiction, the United States has historically first pursued abstinence-only policies. Whether it's sex among teenagers, binge drinking, or trying heroin, the first government-approved model to the alcoholism and addiction is usually "Just Say No!"

In contrast and since the early 1960s, Harm Reductionists have championed sex education to reduce teenage pregnancy, implicitly accepting that teenagers will experiment with sex and that "Just Say No" abstinence programs won't work for many teenagers.

Canada, Britain, and Europe rejected abstinence, mainly because, for them, it just didn't work. Instead, they often allowed experimental programs of Harm Reduction.

PHYSICIANS AND HARM REDUCTION

One prominent doctor in addiction medicine practices Harm Reduction. Dr. Mark Willenbring, director of treatment research from 2004 to 2009 at the National Center for Alcohol Abuse and Alcoholism, treats alcoholism with brief intervention techniques and nonconfrontational therapy, as well as support on drugs to treat depression, anxiety, and other disorders. Such a multifaceted model rejects the disease model and tries to maximize patients' control over their conditions.[4] Purists in AA of the cold-turkey model abhor Willenbring's tolerance of the occasional use of marijuana or a beer.

Small nudges can add up. In one study, each doctor who prescribed opioids to a patient who died from an overdose was sent a letter by authorities in public health notifying him or her of the patient's death and how.[5] Just sending such a letter significantly reduced the number and dosage of subsequent prescriptions for opiates for that physician. Whether it was a Hawthorne

Effect, where the mere fact of someone watching you changes your behavior, or guilt over the death doesn't matter to Harm Reductionists, who just want the deaths to stop.

Physicians who practice harm reduction may run afoul of orthodoxies. Physician Alexander DeLuca, the former chief of addiction medicine at St. Luke's Roosevelt Hospital in New York City, previously ran the Smithers Addiction Treatment and Research Center there. Hired as an abstinence-only advocate, his medical experiences led him to conclude that most addiction medicine should be Harm Reduction. When Dr. DeLuca changed his practice to reflect his experiences, St. Luke's did not rehire him.[6]

As a Harm Reductionist, Dr. DeLuca essentially gave up on seeing addiction as a disease that needed to be cured. If there is no underlying disease, then there is no need to search for a cure. More globally, if gambling, seeing prostitutes, overeating, binge drinking, and texting while driving are not diseases but merely bad behaviors, then those helping people with such problems should focus on modifying the behaviors, not finding the underlying diseases to treat and cure.

HARM REDUCTION, GAMBLING, AND SMOKING

As another example of Harm Reduction, consider gambling, which is a serious problem for a small percentage of people who always chase the Big Win. Harm Reductionists say we should make gambling legal and take it away from the Mafia, which previously ran numbers games as well as illegal betting on horses, fights, and sports contests. In that way, fewer fights and races are fixed.

The decision by the US Supreme Court in 2018 to allow states to pass laws allowing betting on college athletics is approved by Harm Reductionists because it puts everything out in the open and lets governments tax the revenues of widespread gambling on college sports. Social Justice theorists worry that such a change may harm the most vulnerable people who may waste their money on such betting.

Harm Reductionists urge governments to profit from running gambling rather than criminals and then use the profits to reduce problems associated with gambling. In South Africa, where casinos became legal in the twentieth century, a portion of the profits must fund studies and centers to help gambling addicts. Other things can be done, such as taking ATM machines out of casinos and not serving gamblers free alcohol, which reduces their ability to make good judgments.

Harm Reduction has had a long history fighting the terrible effects of worldwide increases in cigarette smoking. A famous debate occurred when a professor of dentistry tried to get cigarette, cigar, and pipe smokers to switch to chewing tobacco, which causes many fewer diseases and deaths than smoked tobacco.[7] The American Cancer Society for a long time took a moralistic, all-or-nothing cold-turkey method, mirroring AA and NA, arguing that smokers should totally quit tobacco in any form and that the only definition of success was total cessation for life.

Decades later, America accepted vaping as a substitute for smoking tobacco, and harm reduction won a great victory (although advocates of the Social Justice model argue that Big Tobacco got behind vaping because it saw new sources of revenue there, especially in enticing teenagers to start vaping; more on this in chapter 11 on legalizing marijuana).

HARM REDUCTION AND AIDS

In 2019, President Trump announced a plan to eradicate HIV/AIDS by 2030.[8] He had already announced the year before that the opioid crisis was a public health emergency. Donald Trump lost a brother to alcoholism in 1981 at the age of forty-three, a death that reportedly affected the president so much that he subsequently never drank alcohol.

The strategy in his 2019 plan targeted forty-eight of the three thousand counties in America where—amazingly but perhaps not surprisingly—50 percent of new HIV infections occur. Two Harm Reduction components of the plan were pre-exposure prophylaxis (PrEP), which is a daily regimen of two oral antiretroviral drugs in a single pill, and needle-exchange programs. The plan targeted pockets of HIV in rural areas of seven states and hoped to reduce new HIV infections by 75 percent in five years.[9]

Harm Reduction's most obvious goal for intravenous drug users is reducing the rate of new hepatitis C infections, with 30,900 new cases in America recorded by the CDC in 2015.[10] Hepatitis C can be cured, but doing so is expensive (and most programs require IV-drug users to be drug free for months before starting treatment). Providing access to clean syringes, sterile water, tourniquets, sharps containers, and filters for IV solutions can dramatically reduce rates of new infection.

ALCOHOLISM AND HARM REDUCTION

With all the news about deaths from prescription opioids and importing fentanyl and heroin, we can easily lose sight of the ongoing toll of alcohol. As noted, on any given weekend, one in six Americans will drink seven drinks in two hours, and afterward, many of them drive home. In 2009, according to the CDC, they caused eleven thousand deaths while driving intoxicated, some of them killing children.[11] The 1.4 million arrests the same year for driving while intoxicated caught only 1 percent of the 147 million episodes of drivers who self-reported that they drove while drunk.[12]

Each year alcoholism causes another fifteen thousand deaths from liver diseases. Alcohol is also a contributing cause in many of our national health problems: heart disease, smoking, and kidney failure. Finally, alcohol almost always hurts people suffering from mental illness.

What does Harm Reduction offer about curbing alcoholism or its bad effects? First, let's call users "heavy drinkers," rather than "alcoholics," because the latter word is so pejorative. Second, let's prevent the worst carnage by emphasizing ways to prevent drunk people from driving.

For example, bars at the University of Georgia at Athens, or at the University of Vermont in Burlington, are allowed to be so close to campus that drunk students need not drive home. At the University of Colorado at Boulder, inebriated students can easily use Uber or Lyft to get home after bars close. The same is true on most college campuses with large student populations.

To actually help the millions of people suffering from alcoholism and AUD, Harm Reduction believes it is necessary to rethink the dominant picture of dealing with these conditions. First, the tough-love approach of intervention may only make individuals hit the road and drive people from their families. Moralizing makes moralizers feel good but does nothing for users, even making drinkers anxious, causing them to want to drink or use drugs again. Dramatic interventions make for good television shows, but unless affected people want to change, they may not work over the long run.

Second, Harm Reduction questions whether the end point of treatment must always be, or even for most people must be, what AA/NA claims: cessation of use for life. Almost everyone realizes that this goal is unrealistic. Worse, it implies that everyone who does not achieve it is a failure. If someone reduces her drinking by 99 percent, why doesn't that count as success? Why focus on the 1 percent and define that as overall failure?

Here is where empirical evaluation of alcohol-cessation programs becomes so important. Because the vast majority of people dependent on alcohol and narcotics can exercise a degree of control over their usage, and because laws and public policy can either discourage or encourage such control, Harm Reductionists say we need to nudge users in the right direction.

Harm Reduction *accepts any method* of getting users to gain more control over their usage and lives. And why should it matter if the goal is to help those who abuse each day? Their families don't care whether AA or Neuroscience or Coping model most helps their loved one: what families want is to stop using money for drugs and use it for food instead.

Harm Reductionists realize that different folks need different methods to learn safe ways to use. Screaming at users in front of others in groups in rehab centers won't work with introverts who fear being around other people. Indeed, introverts avoid AA/NA meetings precisely because they hate the idea of being humiliated in groups. By contrast, some people hate being alone and need the support of a group to change: they can recover *only* in a group. To stay clean, they may need to go to a group meeting every day.

Third, Harm Reduction disagrees with AA/NA that users don't need medication substitution to kick drugs. As writer and recovering alcoholic Leslie Jamison notes at the end of her book, "For much of the second half of the twentieth century, many rehabs steeped in twelve-step recovery believed that medication-assisted treatment compromised sobriety. It's as if medication became a sign of moral failure, a sign that someone was effectively still using."[13]

One great insight of studies of the brain is that users initially chase a high, then get decreasing returns on their usage, in other words, less and less of a high. After a period of usage, the pattern flips, where, instead of chasing a high, users are avoiding the misery of withdrawal. It is exactly that point where most addiction-therapists agree that the user must get some medication to make him feel less miserable when he's not using his drug of choice.[14]

Thus, most drug-dependent users will need buspirone, methadone, or benzodiazepines to help their cravings stop; Harm Reductionists are even okay with substituting high-dose marijuana for opiates because at least the former is legal in some states.

However, drug substitution for treating addiction is highly controversial and not a settled action. Cocaine was introduced in medicine as a non-addicting drug substitution for heroin. Oxycontin was marketed as a faintly addicting substitute for traditional narcotics and heroin. And as we shall see in chapter 11, high-dosage recreational marijuana with 90 percent THC concentrations may be just as addicting as opiates.

Kantians and Narcotics Anonymous would stress that Harm Reduction strategies must really reduce harms. Just switching affected uses from one addicting drug to another doesn't do much good.

Amazingly, some users don't need anything to moderate their usage, other than exercise and friends. But these people tend to be in their mid-thirties and with otherwise good life prospects. This is an example of the previously discussed "maturing out."

For alcohol, we know that drinkers get less drunk on a full stomach than an empty one (which is why abusers drink on empty stomachs *before* eating rather than *with* the meal or *after* the meal). We know that hard whiskey makes people drunk faster than light beer. We know that two shots of tequila make a 120-pound woman drunk faster than a 280-pound man. To reduce these problems, Harm Reduction teaches people to eat before they drink, to switch from hard whiskey to light wine or light beer, and to discourage women from matching the drinking of men.

Public policy can follow Harm Reduction and lessen the possibility of drunk driving: Some cities make bartenders and owners of bars responsible for letting people drive away while falling-down drunk. Put breath-analyzers on cars of people convicted of DWIs, such that they can't drive with alcohol-saturated breath.

HARM REDUCTION, NALOXONE, AND OPIATE ADDICTION

Cities such as Vancouver in Canada have offered addicts safe clinics for injection, giving them clean needles and supervised injection, such that if the substance is heavily cut with fentanyl and the user overdoses, naloxone (trade name Narcan) can be administered on site to save the user's life.

Naloxone, an "opioid antagonist," counters the effects of opioids on the central nervous system and breathing, allowing the victim to breathe normally and avoid brain damage from anoxia. When injected intravenously, it acts within two minutes; when injected intramuscularly, five minutes.[15] If the victim is breathing, it can also be given as a nasal spray. In some communities in Massachusetts and the Northeast, where many people die each year of overdoses, Harm Reduction advocates successfully campaigned for every first responder to have naloxone on hand. They wanted families of users to also have it, as well as partners of addicted people.

Ohio has been one of the hardest-hit states in America: In 2018, 4,800 people died there of overdoses. Dayton and Cincinnati were epicenters of such deaths. In response and with the urging of Harm Reduction advocates, officials in these cities supplied 37,000 units of naloxone to first responders and counselors, dropping overdose deaths by one-third.[16] Rather than eight calls a day about overdoses, emergency crews sometimes had no calls. Dayton had similar success with flooding its citizens with naloxone: it reduced deaths from overdoses from more than 500 a year to less than 250.[17]

Several states now require physicians writing prescriptions for opiates to simultaneously write prescriptions for naloxone.[18] If such a policy went national in America, drug companies would sell an additional 48 million doses of naloxone.

As another example of implementing Harm Reduction consistently, consider making naloxone available without prescription. In fourteen states in America, those who distribute naloxone to ordinary families without a prescription break the law, making some refuse to do so. In another thirty-six states, it's illegal to carry naloxone on one's person without a prescription. Nurses who carry naloxone in their purses as Good Samaritans can be denied life insurance because the insurers think they're using the drugs on themselves rather than trying to save lives.[19]

Although well intentioned, these strategies are not without their critics. As with previous battles over harm-reduction strategies, critics see distribution of naloxone as encouraging bad behavior, especially higher and higher doses of heroin or fentanyl-laced oxycodone. So long as someone is nearby to save them, won't users take bigger risks? So long as first responders rush to revive unresponsive users, why not risk the biggest dosage for the greatest high?

NEW HARM-REDUCTION STRATEGIES TO REDUCING DEATHS

Various provinces and states hit hardest by the epidemic have tried new ideas. The province of British Columbia in 2019 is experimenting with giving addicted people matchstick-sized implants of buprenorphine, similar to the Norplant implants for birth control.[20] As a medication-substitution strategy, the implant in the upper arm releases a little of the drug each day, reducing craving. The danger is that addicts can still use illicit drugs, piling an injection on top of the daily dose from the implant.

The pioneering Australian physician George O'Neil has implanted a device that releases a little naltrexone into stomachs of addicted people and thus blocks the effects of opioids.[21] The implants are legal in Australia but not in North America.

In 2014, Vermont used its extensive system of social services and Catamount Health Coverage to reduce waiting time for treatment for opioid addiction. It supplied users with methadone or buprenorphine to reduce cravings and paired users with counselors and support groups.[22]

But five years later, the number of opioid fatalities still rose: they rose more than 40 percent from 2015, from 74 to 110 deaths a year for Vermonters.[23] But without these strategies, there may have been even more deaths.

In 2019, Kentucky had fifty "syringe service centers," which also gave out naloxone and referrals for counseling and social services.[24] Pennsylvania, whose neighborhood of Kensington in Philadelphia had become a national mecca for scoring cheap heroin (see chapter 10), made naloxone available to anyone without a prescription; as a result, in December 2018, it gave away more than six thousand naloxone kits.

HARM REDUCTION AND SAFE-INJECTION SITES

A controversial proposal today of the Harm Reduction Coalition is supervised, safe-injection sites (also called "drug consumption rooms") for people using needles to inject narcotics.[25] In 2018, a report in Washington State recommended establishment of two supervised injection sites, which, it said,

offer a supervised place for hygienic consumption of drugs in a non-judgmental environment free from stigma, while providing low-barrier access to on-site health services and screenings, referrals, and linkages to behavioral health and other supportive services (for example, housing).[26]

In 2015, the Harm Reduction Coalition held a conference with experts in international law enforcement and public health to understand local dynamics opposing safe-injection sites for drug consumption. The result was a landmark document, "Alternates to Public Injection," which claimed that IV-drug users who used these sites: (1) reduced or eliminated needle sharing, reducing rates of new infections of HIV and hepatitis; (2) gained access to medical and social services, especially drug treatment programs; (3) had not one fatal overdose; (4) did not encourage drug usage or young people to start; and (5) decreased crime and public nuisances after start of these programs.[27]

People living around such sites reject the last claim. To avoid this problem, a van offering clean needles in Tacoma, Washington, travels to different parking lots on different days, to avoid having users camp at any geographical site.

Giving users access to medical treatment and social services at such sites is controversial in that they may use such services not to cease usage, but rather to manage acute problems such as infections.

According to the international Harm Reduction Coalition, about ninety safe-injection sites operate in Australia, Europe, and Canada. They provide alternatives to restrooms of fast-food shops, public parks, or libraries, where used needles can be discarded and found by children. Legal self-injection sites mostly exist in northern Europe, where approximately sixty operate in thirty-six cities.[28]

Safe-injection sites are most effective in reducing rates of transmission of infectious diseases and reducing rates of overdose deaths. In general, they do not reduce the numbers of substance abusers and, when free and offered, usually do not get most substance abusers into treatment. In Seattle, although not legal, about a dozen safe-injection sites exist and are tolerated by law enforcement officials.[29]

Objections to such sites fall along two lines, both with historical pedigrees. The first is NIMBY ("not in my back yard"), in which local citizens object to attracting drug users to their neighborhood. Their concern has been verified historically, as drug users show up early before a center opens and, after injecting, don't go far. A common falsehood about drug users is that they are zombie-stoned all day and night, but, in fact, most have significant time between injections when they look to eat, find money to pay for injections, and do normal activities. But owners of local houses and businesses don't want hundreds, or thousands, of addicted people roaming their neighborhoods, much less camping there.

The second objection to self-injection sites is that such sites either encourage drug usage or tolerate something that law and public policy should not tolerate.

This objection matches the one made when students in the mid-1980s at Yale University proposed a site where local IV-drug users could safely inject. In 1988, pioneer Dave Purchase started such a program in Tacoma, Washington, to prevent infections with HIV, and it later switched to preventing deaths from overdoses.

The US government long opposed needle-swap programs to reduce new infections of HIV and hepatitis. After thirty years, it realized that HIV and needle sharing are not going away, and, perhaps more important, the costs of treating infections of HIV and hepatitis are exorbitant, so it has allowed such programs to operate. Three hundred twenty programs now function in areas of heavy usage, such as where southern Ohio meets Kentucky. The program in Tacoma celebrated its thirtieth year in 2018.[30] Harm Reductionists wonder whether it will take the same government forty years to embrace safe-injection sites.

Another controversial proposal by an advocate of Harm Reduction comes from Tim Lahey, a physician and bioethicist at the Dartmouth-Hitchcock

Medical Center in New Hampshire, whose state ranks in the top five for opioid deaths.[31] Almost every day, he and his medical staff try "to save a young person dying from infectious complications of injection drug use."[32]

When hospitalized for liver problems from hepatitis, or infections of heart valves, users miss their customary drugs. If family and friends cannot visit (and cannot bring drugs), and patients are not allowed to go anywhere private where they can shoot up, users start to perceive hospitals and medical staff as jailors. Rather than employing guards to prevent addicted patients from injecting drugs, Dr. Lahey proposes safe rooms in overburdened hospitals where patients can inject and avoid conflicts with hospital staff, similar to some VA hospitals where smokers addicted to nicotine can smoke away from oxygen and other patients.

PHILADELPHIA'S KENSINGTON AREA AND ZURICH'S "PLATZSPITZ PARK"

In 2019, the city of Philadelphia battled the US Department of Justice over establishing a safe-injection site in Kensington, a neighborhood of South Philadelphia, which attracted many opiate-using people.[33] A nonprofit group, Safehouse, wanted to start a site there to lower the high rate of overdoses. San Francisco had already legalized such a safe house, but Governor Jerry Brown vetoed it.

The Justice Department under the Trump administration opposed the program, arguing that it would encourage usage. The US district attorney for the area said, "Normalizing use of deadly drugs like heroin and fentanyl is not the answer to solving the opioid epidemic."

The Justice Department sued in federal court for an injunction against Safehouse, appealing to the Controlled Substances Act that made it illegal under federal law to manage a site for the "purpose of unlawfully using a controlled substance."[34] Safehouse retorted that it was imperative to save lives, not save neighborhoods or stop substance abusers from using.

Rod Rosenstein, then deputy attorney general of the United States, strenuously opposed other proposals for safe-injection sites. Representing the US government, he cited the constant risks to staff when users inject fentanyl, which "can be up to fifty times more powerful than heroin."[35] Second, he accepted the NIMBY objection by stating that safe-injection sites harm the communities in which they are embedded, attracting many more addicts than would normally be there. Third, "injection sites normalize drug use and facilitate addiction by sending a powerful message to teenagers that government thinks illegal drugs can be used safely."

Finally, Rosenstein claimed that less than 10 percent of those using safe-injection sites in Vancouver, Portugal, or Europe, even when it's free and easily available, ever entered treatment. Rosenstein implied that this was because most addicted people don't want to change, and if that is a fact, then making it safer to keep using opiates is not good public policy.

Indeed, some evidence exists that safe-injection sites allow drug users to get bigger highs because they no longer fear dying. And with cheap fentanyl replacing cheap heroin on the streets, the risk of dying has grown.

Critics of Harm Reduction despised what happened in Kensington. Due to local police tolerance, dealers operated in the open and gave out free samples. Streets abounded with people smoking meth or crack, even openly sticking needles in their arms. Adverse selection drew addicted people from up and down the East Coast, who heard that cheap heroin could be had in Kensington along with tolerance for open usage. Within months, hundreds of addicted people flocked to the area. As the *New York Times* reported in 2018:

> [Kensington] is known for having both the cheapest and purest heroin in the region and is a major supplier for dealers in Delaware, New Jersey and Maryland. For years, the heroin being sold in Kensington was pure enough to snort, but that summer, it was mixed with unpredictable amounts of fentanyl. In Philadelphia, deaths related to fentanyl had increased by 95 percent in the past year.
>
> Philadelphia County has the highest overdose rate of any of the 10 most populous counties in America. The city's Department of Health estimates that 75,000 residents are addicted to heroin and other opioids, and each day, many of them commute to Kensington to buy drugs. The neighborhood is part of the largest cluster of overdose deaths in the city. In 2017, 236 people fatally overdosed there.[36]

Philosopher George Santayana famously wrote that those ignorant of the past are condemned to repeat its mistakes. For critics of Harm Reduction, Philadelphia is repeating the mistakes of Zurich, Switzerland, which in the 1990s tolerated an open-air drug market in its Platzspitz Park.[37] At one point, as many as three thousand drug addicts a day entered this park, and the number of heroin users buying there spiked ten times from three thousand in 1975 to thirty thousand in 1992. The *New York Times* famously dubbed it "Needle Park."[38]

Advocates for Harm Reduction reply that the Swiss made key mistakes: They decriminalized heroin but did not offer addicts therapy. They did not offer therapy involving drug substitution, nor did they establish safe places to use other than the park.

The Drug Policy Foundation champions Harm Reduction. Its president, Arnold Trebach, wrote in 1992 about this experiment:

> The drug free-for-all that flourished at Platzspitz was the result of an unplanned local compromise not representative of any drug policy reform proposals.
>
> What developed at Needle Park was the worst of both worlds. The park was an island of limited decriminalization in the midst of one of the most harshly prohibitionist societies in Europe. Platzspitz became Needle Park only gradually, as addicts congregate [there]. Local authorities tolerated drug activities . . . to ghettoize the drug problem.
>
> This was not an ideal arrangement, but the Swiss at least attempted to respond to the serious problems they faced as a result of strict across-the-board prohibition. Unfortunately, Needle Park was a half-measure from the start, and many predictable problems were not dealt with.
>
> Until about two years ago, the strategy was simply for the police to be hands-off within the park. There was no public health planning; no controls over drugs sold; no age restrictions; indeed, no controls of any sort. Thus, to call Needle Park an experiment is dubious. It was not a social policy chosen as best from a range of proposals.[39]

Critics point to Platzspitz as an example of what happens when heroin is decriminalized and users are allowed to inject in public. Trebach claims nobody wants to decriminalize *public* use of heroin ("no serious reform advocates want public drug use. Most comprehensive options include harsh sanctions for those who use drugs in public or work or drive intoxicated"). Some safe-injection sites work well if well planned and located. "Three crucial examples are Liverpool, Amsterdam, and methadone programs within the United States. All . . . reduced crime, reduced drug abuse and controlled the spread of AIDS among the individuals involved." Decriminalize, yes, Trebach argues, but make users inject in safe, private places.

With Platzspitz Park, the surrounding area predictably saw huge increases in prostitution, discarded needles, and crime. In 1992, the Swiss offered addicts methadone and followed even more radically in 1994 by offering legal prescriptions for heroin. To get them out of the park, some addicted Swiss citizens even got public housing.

Years of public debate ensued in Switzerland about the best method of dealing with addicted citizens. In 2008, the Swiss voted to make non-punitive approaches legal. By 2017, about 80 percent of addicts in Switzerland were in substitution therapy (90 percent getting methadone, 10 percent getting heroin).

Today, Platzspitz Park is a pleasant park without addicts and filled with normal citizens reading on lunch breaks and kids playing. To date, no other country has followed Switzerland, either in tolerating an area where users can openly buy and use drugs or in publicly funding drug-substitution therapy. In particular, no other European country allows heroin to be prescribed. That option, which is a Harm Reduction maneuver to reduce crime and prostitution, remains highly controversial. Predictably, it is seen by critics as enabling addiction to heroin and taking away any incentive to kick the habit.

CANADIAN HARM REDUCTION

Canada has aggressively tried to use harm-reduction techniques to stem its rising number of opioid-associated deaths, especially in its western province of British Columbia, where 1,854 Canadians died from overdoses in the eighteen months between January 2016 and July 2017.

British Columbia allows some things that would be considered radical in America. First, it allows for a safe-injection site, Insite, in east Vancouver, so if users overdose there, they can be immediately revived by trained attendants. Insite has operated since 2003, although it has been subjected to several legal challenges.[40]

Second, the Insite facility in east Vancouver allows users to quickly test their street drugs for contamination before injection. The facility uses the same drug-testing technology pioneered in Europe at dance festivals to test ecstasy (street name Molly), a necessity that became apparent in the same province when a star pre-med student took "Sally" thinking it was "Molly" and died.[41]

The Insite facility also came about partly because some addicted people in Vancouver called 911 to summon first responders before they shot up, wanting first responders around in case their stuff had too much fentanyl and would kill them. When they felt safe, they (or their partner) told first responders they had mistakenly called.[42] With the new Insite center, such misuse of first responders in Vancouver vanished.

British Columbia also tries to avoid short-term shock therapies for users, which are aimed at rapid detoxification but associated with relapses and deaths; instead it focuses on long-term solutions. Thus, the province provides opioid-agonist drugs (bupremorphine and methadone) to most citizens free of charge. Finally, the province offers slow-release naloxone and experimental programs that allow users to take naloxone home.

PORTUGAL

Portugal in 2001 decriminalized use of all drugs, even heroin and cocaine.[43] Twenty years before, it had the highest rate in Europe of HIV infection in IV-drug users. At that time, as many as 100,000 Portuguese were addicted to heroin, resulting in two thousand new HIV infections a year. Thus, it avoids the harms of incarcerating thousands of people and the deaths and contraction of STDs of thousands more.

One new Harm Reduction strategy in Portugal was to allow drug users to swap dirty syringes and needles for clean new supplies not at special houses or roving vans (as in Tacoma, Washington) but at pharmacy counters. As a result, each year between 1995 and 1999, pharmacies in Portugal supplied three million drug kits to drug users.[44]

According to *New York Times* columnist Nicholas Kristoff, "If the US could achieve Portugal's (low) death rate from drugs, we would save one life every 10 minutes. We would save almost as many lives as are now lost to guns and car accidents combined."[45] The number of fatal drug overdoses dropped 85 percent in Portugal between 2001 and 2017, giving it the lowest rate in Europe for both overdoses and new, drug-related HIV infections.

Critics say that Portugal's plan wouldn't work in America because Portugal resisted allowing physicians to overprescribe opioids, while America did not. In addition, Portugal has free, easy treatment for opioid addiction and a social safety net that helps drug users live.

However, not everything is great in Portugal. Either because of increased honesty on the part of drug users or because the numbers actually changed, after decades of its new policy, more people than ever in Portugal report using cocaine, marijuana, ecstasy, and heroin.[46] This fact somewhat mirrors what happened in Vermont, where extensive medical support and drug-substitution therapy in its comprehensive Catamount medical system did not reduce fatal overdoses, although more Portuguese did enter free government treatment.

MOTHERS: ANY SAFE LEVELS FOR DRINKING AND OPIATES?

Drinking/Using during Pregnancy

One of the great, ongoing debates concerns whether any use of alcohol or opiates is safe for fetuses during pregnancy. The body of medical evidence seems to say, "No amount of alcohol or opiates is safe for fetuses during pregnancy."[47]

Given that almost half of pregnant women in Ireland admit to binge drinking during pregnancy, one begins to understand the worldwide danger of drugs and opiates to newborns. A 2018 study showed that 10 percent of pregnant American women drink alcohol, resulting in as many as 5 percent of their babies born with fetal alcohol spectrum disorder, which now occurs more frequently than autism.[48]

How much low IQ, ADHD, autism, and personality disorder might be caused by substance abuse during pregnancy? Because we can't do controlled experiments with pregnant women, we will never know, but it's frightening to speculate, especially because some scholars think the most damage occurs very early in pregnancy.

Of course, this makes it very hard on pregnant women, especially young women who have become accustomed to using alcohol to relax. Can we really ask them, once they decide to get pregnant, to abstain from alcohol and all serious drugs for nine months?

Breastfeeding and Drugs

The Centers for Disease Control says that one drink a day for a breastfeeding mother is not known to be harmful to the baby if the mother waits at least two hours before nursing. However, longer waits are required for safety with a higher number of drinks—for example, four to five hours after two drinks and six to eight hours after three drinks. However, "exposure to alcohol above moderate levels through breast milk could be damaging to an infant's development, growth, and sleep patterns."[49]

Breastfeeding is also not recommended by CDC for pregnant women on opiates.[50] The worry is that even brief exposure to opiates, either in gestation or with breastfeeding, may expose children to lifelong impairment in cognitive, emotional and motivational abilities. The truth is that we do not know the harm that these substances may cause to fetuses and neonates, and because we can't do randomized controlled trials to prove things one way or the other, we should assume they are unsafe.

Neonatal Abstinence Syndrome

Neonatal Abstinence Syndrome (NAS) is a tragic condition well known to neonatologists resulting from exposure of fetuses during gestation to drugs. Before the recent epidemic of opiates and heroin, neonatologists knew the dangers of women smoking and drinking while pregnant. Fetal alcohol syndrome resulted, and, for smoking mothers, the infant suffered withdrawal from nicotine. Today, they worry about fetuses being dependent on heroin, oxycodone, methadone, benzodiazepines, and buprenorphine.

A large ethical question looms about how to best manage the baby's withdrawal from such drugs. Such babies produce distinctive cries and during withdrawal may suffer seizures, tremors, extreme irritability, apnea, and convulsions. Some doctors would wean the infants from the drugs, while others urge abstinence and cold-turkey quitting. If the learning approach is correct, the infant should not suffer in the same way from withdrawal as adults because the infant has not learned to use drugs in any way to cope with life's problems. However, the infant does seem to suffer physical withdrawal. This is a special example of the issue known in philosophy as the "problem of other minds." In this case, we can't get inside the mind of the baby.

HARM REDUCTION AND FAMILIES

To their credit, both Alcoholics Anonymous and Narcotics Anonymous developed support groups for families touched by alcoholism and addiction. In many ways, such groups practice Harm Reduction, because they help families support recovery while also setting limits when the relative doesn't want to recover.

WHAT OTHER MODELS GET WRONG

Harm Reduction opposes the implicit moralism in the Kantian model. Everyone may theoretically be free to not try opiates, or to kick them cold turkey, but some people are freer than others to do so: those with supportive families, good health coverage, and good jobs have things that many addicted people lack.

Libertarians seem especially harsh in criticizing addicted people for their choices. Such criticism will likely just make people want to escape more into drugs. It may satisfy the one who is criticizing, making him feel better about his life and choices, but it doesn't help anyone else.

Harm Reductionists say they can't wait for neuroscientists and geneticists to discover the exact causes of addiction and, more important, how to reverse these causes at a deep level. In the meantime, Harm Reductionists deal with everyday needs, just trying to keep addicted people alive.

THE HARM OF TOTAL AND RAPID WITHDRAWAL PROGRAMS

If we have learned anything from the biology of alcoholism and addiction, it is that the bodies of most people won't tolerate quick withdrawal. For some people, total withdrawal is just not realistic.

But a whole other class of patients exist, patients who have a legitimate, perhaps lifelong need for relief for pain, such as someone who had his spine crushed in an industrial accident and was left with damaged nerves. Among the patients of the infamous Dr. Jack Kevorkian, some of the saddest cases of people who came to him for help in dying were patients not with terminal diseases but with intractable pain.

Because of worries about opioid addiction, in 2016 the CDC issued guidelines to physicians treating patients dependent on opioids, the most important of which was a recommendation against prescribing opioids except for palliative care for dying patients.[51] Unfortunately, according to three hundred physicians in addiction medicine, too many physicians interpreted CDC's recommendation as a *requirement* and either stopped prescribing or drastically tapered their prescribed dosages.

Forced tapering may harm patients in chronic pain, according to Stefan Kertesz, MD, at the University of Alabama in Birmingham, a leader in the movement to resist interpreting CDC's guidelines as mandatory. As there may be as many as eighteen million patients in this condition, forced tapering is a big deal for many patients and their physicians. This fact was painfully discovered personally by a bioethicist at Johns Hopkins who became addicted to oxycodone after a motorcycle accident and who got little help in weaning himself from the drugs.[52]

Again, Harm Reduction is not purist. Its goal is not necessarily to have all patients off all drugs. It accepts the fact that bad luck will wreck some people's lives and leave them in terrible pain. Medicine is lucky that if it can't cure these patients, it can help relieve their pain with opioids, even for life. For some, a fentanyl patch can give them a few hours of relief. Harm Reductionists are fine with that.

CRITICISMS OF HARM REDUCTION FROM OTHER MODELS

Both Kantians and Alcoholics Anonymous see Harm Reduction as amoral and relativistic, encouraging such behaviors as here to stay. Notice that the Portuguese do not claim that they've cured addicts or stopped them from lifetime usage—only that they've saved them from fatal overdoses or getting hepatitis or AIDS.

Social Justice champions see Harm Reduction as putting a bandage on a hemorrhaging patient. If North America is being flooded with opiates and cheap, fentanyl-laced heroin, what good are small efforts to prevent fatalities and addiction? The head of the snake must be cut off, rather than just starving the snake or enticing it not to bite humans.

From different perspectives, the Neuroscience and Genetics models would also see Harm Reduction as putting bandages on the symptoms of an underlying biological disease. However, champions of the Coping model are most likely to agree with many of the goals of Harm Reduction, especially in helping individuals to control the worst effects of their behavior.

CONCLUSIONS

Harm Reduction won't appeal to everyone, but it has its place. Even if addiction is seen as a chronic, often relapsing condition, the goal need not be lifelong abstinence—merely reduction in the number and intensity of relapses. Relapses can occur without fatalities or transmission of STDs. Relapses can occur without loss of a job or driver's license.

To be most effective, Harm Reduction will need to work at different levels: in personal changes by the user, in support with medication substitution and groups, in adequate coverage for reimbursement for the previous support, and in high-level public policy that supports safe houses and distribution of naloxone. In America, the Social Justice model is also correct that unless the oversupply of Oxycontin and cheap heroin stops, more Band-aids won't stop the epidemic.

Summary of the Harm Reduction Model

Underlying cause: Searching for an underlying cause of addiction does not matter; there is an urgent need to help victims now; we may never discover the true cause of alcoholism or addiction, and we cannot wait for the answer; we must mitigate harms now. The very idea that every compulsive bad behavior has an underlying cause may be a mistake.

Treatment: Focus on reducing harms extrinsic to using substances; teach new behavior; decriminalize drugs; expand access and kinds of treatment.

Other models: They allow harm and death to mount while focusing on quixotic quests to discover the true cause of alcoholism/addiction. Or they engage in unhelpful moralism.

Responsibility: Users can be taught and nudged to make better choices; emphasizing personal responsibility is one tool among others for Harm Reduction and will work with some.

Family matters: Alcoholism and addiction always affect more than one person: they affect partners, children, parents, friends, and colleagues. Those around the addicted person can learn to limit the damage to themselves and set limits to how much they give. Treatment should help not only the substance abuser but also those in significant relationships with him. Relatives of substance abusers may be traumatized and harmed as much as the person with the disorder. In some cases, the best way to reduce the most harm may not be to help the substance abuser but to help her family. After all, it is better that only one person's life is wasted rather than five. Many families today are enmeshed with their adult children and find it difficult to extricate themselves from an addicted child. Probably the most difficult decision of all is to draw a firm line and stay firm, even at risk of estrangement. But some families need to do this or risk total destruction from one addicted relative. Moreover, relatives should not be forgotten in formulating public policy about treatment for addiction and alcoholic. If the substance abuser recovers, that does not mean the family has recovered and doesn't fear a relapse.

WRITTEN IN THE DNA

I was only seven years old, but I knew, with a fundamental-
ist's fervor, that the party was potentially lethal. Not because
of my [Native American] mother's and father's actions, but
because of their inattentions. They were alcoholics who'd
get what they laughingly called bottle-blind, as in "I was so
bottle-blind that I didn't even realize I'd driven off the road
until I woke up with a pine tree branch sticking through the
car windshield about four inches from my nose." That's
what my father said—or approximately what he said—after
his eleventh or nineteenth or twenty-seventh drunken car
wreck.

—Sherman Alexie, *You Don't Have to Say You Love Me*

According to the National Institute on Alcohol Abuse and Alcoholism,
Alcohol Abuse Disorder (AUD) runs in families and "genetics certainly
influence our likelihood of developed AUD."[1] Although the Institute states
that a specific, single gene for alcoholism does not exist, it still claims that
"research shows that genes are responsible for about half of the risk for AUD."
Mark Willenbring, director of treatment research for this Institute from 2004
to 2009, claims even more powerfully that 60 percent of alcohol and drug
dependence is caused by genes.[2] Presumably, genetic inheritance would also
underlie Opiate Use Disorder (OUD).

As an example of how genes may run in families to cause substance abuse,
consider tech wizard Colin Kroll, who founded Vine, a six-second video-
sharing platform bought by Twitter in 2012 for $30 million. After that, Kroll
created Intermedia Labs, which created the popular game-show app HQ
Trivia.

Colin Kroll may have inherited not only high intelligence but also something else: genes for alcoholism. His grandfather and father both struggled for years with alcoholism and his uncle, after diving into a lake while drunk, became partially paralyzed.[3]

After Kroll received millions from Twitter's purchase of Vine, he became addicted to alcohol and cocaine, eventually graduating to heroin. In December 2017, his girlfriend found him, heroin and cocaine nearby, in his apartment in New York City, dead at age thirty-four. Ruled an accidental overdose, the heroin near his dead body had been laced with fentanyl.

Did Colin Kroll's genes set him up for early death? Once his life took a downward turn, did genes predestine him to heavy use of alcohol and hard drugs? Did the same genetic pull affect his father, grandfather, and uncle? If drugs and alcohol tempt everyone, are some more tempted than others, right from the first use?

Paul Thomas, a physician running a clinic for addicted youth, thinks so: "Based on studies that looked at addiction in siblings, particularly twins, it appears that 50 to 60 percent of addiction is hereditary."[4] He opens his book by admitting that he and his wife are recovering, respectively, from alcoholism and addiction, and that his three biological children have struggled with substance abuse, implying a genetic basis for it all.[5]

Dr. Thomas suggests that people who are worried about alcoholism and addiction should have their single-nucleotide polymorphisms tested by 23andMe for vulnerability to alcoholism and addiction. He states that such vulnerabilities do not fatalistically decree one's future and stresses that knowledge of them can be powerful. For example, he refers to his wife's physician, who had alcoholism in his family history, but who—because he feared his inherited risk—never had even one drink.[6] President Donald Trump, after his older brother Fred died young from alcoholism, appears to have reacted the same way.[7]

Some organizations, such as Recovery Village, claim that "children with parents who are alcoholics are anywhere from three to four times more likely than their peers to be addicted to alcohol."[8] Researchers in genetics believe that vulnerability to addiction is "moderately to highly heritable" (more on exactly what this means later). They point to the Virginia Twin Study, which revealed that social factors determine use of alcohol and marijuana in early adolescence, but in young and middle adulthood, genetic factors become important.[9] These researchers conclude:

> Like other complex diseases, such as obesity, diabetes, cancer, coronary heart
> disease, and AIDS, the addictions are strongly influenced by genetic background

and also profoundly influenced by lifestyle and individual choices. Although addictions show no clear pattern of Mendelian inheritance and their complexity is poorly understood, on the basis of their moderate to high heritability it is evident that they are strongly influenced by inherited functional variations, and identification of these alleles is key to understanding the puzzle of causality.[10]

According to the National Council on Alcoholism and Drug Dependence (NCADD), a family history of alcoholism or addiction strongly predicts similar problems in children:

> Research has shown conclusively that family history of alcoholism or drug addiction is in part genetic *and not just the result of the family environment* (emphasis added). . . . millions of Americans are living proof. Plain and simple, alcoholism and drug dependence run in families.[11]

For thirty years, the National Institute on Alcohol Abuse and Alcoholism funded a study of the genetic causes of alcoholism: the Collaborative Study on Genetics of Alcoholism (COGA).[12] COGA covers almost eighteen thousand people over several generations in more than two thousand families in six clusters in Connecticut; Indiana; Brooklyn, New York; Iowa; San Diego, California; and St. Louis, Missouri. Its diagnosis of alcohol dependence uses several tools (DSM-III-R, Feighner, ICD-10) "as well as examination of medical records and direct assessment of people using the Semi-Structured Assessment for Genetics of Alcoholism (SSAGA)." It also keeps samples of the DNA of everyone for potential later analysis.

Some addictionologists believe that for some individuals, genetic predispositions may be as important as, or more important than, the claim in the Neuroscience model that repeated exposure to a drug creates an acquired disease of the brain. For example, Carlton Erickson, with forty-five years of research on addiction as a professor of pharmacology, believes that for some people, susceptibility to alcoholism or addiction *"is in the brain at birth"* (my emphasis).

According to this model of addiction, genetic vulnerability *causes* the disease when the brain is exposed to the drug.[13] So some geneticists think the neuroscientists just come late to the real, underlying cause—namely, the genetic predisposition that makes a brain so receptive to being changed by alcohol and hard drugs.

In this model, whether addiction occurs with one use, within the first year of use, or only after years of use depends on how the genes are expressed by environmental cofactors and whether, say, one or two copies of alcohol-predisposing genes or addiction-predisposing genes are inherited (more on this soon).

Genes can also be correlated with good things, such as longevity. For example, a well-known study at Einstein Medical College's Institute for Aging Research of five hundred elderly people between the ages of 85 and 112 discovered a high preponderance of Ashkenazi Jews who survived past age 95. They had the "Methuselah" variation in a gene governing insulin-like growth factor 1 receptor (IGF1R).[14] Thus genes may determine not only who dies early but also who lives the longest, regardless of upbringing, diet, family, or culture. If that is so, they may also determine who becomes addicted and, in the reverse, who, once addicted, later matures and stops using.

ALCOHOL AND THE FIRST PEOPLES

Historically, although many white settlers tried to live peacefully with Native Americans, other war-prone, racist newcomers, eager for more good land, inevitably started wars, from the massacre of the Pequots at Mystic, Connecticut, in 1636 to the vast French and Indian War of 1763, and then on to later slaughters west of the Mississippi River.[15] In almost all the cases, solemn promises made by the US government were broken and Native Americans were then evicted from their ancestral lands.

In more peaceful times, powerful people have always used alcohol and drugs such as opium to control vulnerable people. Traders in North America deliberately used alcohol to harm Native Americans (now often called "First Peoples"). Very soon, traders realized that many First Peoples were highly susceptible to alcoholism and, when drunk, made bad trades. As early as 1777, traders often plied them with a barrel of rum before trading began.

Nor has the legacy of alcoholism disappeared into ancient history. Alcoholism continues to plague the First Peoples today. Native Americans living around reservations have a very high incidence of maternal-fetal alcohol syndrome, where babies are born dependent on alcohol and where their intelligence and personalities have been damaged by heavy exposure to alcohol in the womb.

Older Native American women, seeing the carnage in the men and youth around them, are the most likely to abstain. They understand their risk of becoming alcoholics and understand the likely damage. But is the prevalent alcoholism and addiction cultural, genetic, or neither? Consider the following famous case in bioethics.

A CASE STUDY OF GENETICS AND ALCOHOLISM: ERNIE CROWFEATHER

In 1968 in Ellensburg, Washington, after a weekend of binge drinking, Ernie, a twenty-six-year-old half-Sioux, half-white man, entered his hospital's emergency room, coughing up yellow sputum and blood, with pain in his left kidney. Ernie needed experimental hemodialysis, which at the time was a brand-new procedure and not covered by insurance. Eventually, physicians found Ernie a dialysis machine by fabricating a research protocol specific to Ernie at another hospital.

However, Ernie did not want to stop drinking, so he missed several appointments for dialysis. During the thirty months that Ernie was on dialysis, physicians rescued him several times in ways they never did for healthier, more compliant patients. Why? In part because Ernie was half-Sioux, in part because he was charming, in part because he was what his sister called "a con man."

Consistently noncompliant, Ernie not only kept on drinking but also, during his last months, used narcotics and barbiturates and refused to learn home dialysis. Physicians spent a lot of money and time on Ernie for treatment he did not want, while other anonymous people died for lack of treatment, 95 percent of whom would have done well on home dialysis.[16]

Nephrologists in Seattle tried repeatedly to get Ernie Crowfeather to stop drinking and to adopt healthy living habits so he could live on hemodialysis. But he wouldn't.

Ernie's final day came on July 29, 1971. Eleven days before, after months of having his veins cut and recut painfully for dialysis, after money raised for him had run out, and to get money for more treatment, he robbed a Hilton Hotel. Arrested immediately and released for dialysis, he never went to jail. A week later, he intercepted a check for $2,000 meant to pay his bills, cashed it, and paid off some debts.

He then checked into a remote motel (as he told his sister later) "to drink myself into oblivion." Missing his scheduled dialysis appointments, his friends began searching for him to no avail. In his final phone call, he said, "I'm so alone."

Ernie's sister figured out where he was and raced to find him. When she did, he was sick from having missed dialysis for several days and from his drinking. She got him alive to the local hospital, but he died that night.[17]

DID ERNIE'S GENES MAKE HIM DRINK?

Some geneticists firmly believe that destructive drinking such as Ernie Crow-feather's stems not from free will but from his inherited genes as a Native American. In a 2003 study in *Human Genetics* of 582 adult members of a Southwest Native American tribe, 85 percent of males over age thirty-five met "the DSM-III-R criteria for alcohol-dependence at some point in their lives" and nearly 65 percent of them had engaged in binge drinking.[18] Nevertheless, all these Native American males also experienced the kind of toxic effects that make other people sick from drinking alcohol. So why did these Native Americans keep drinking?

Exactly what is occurring with genes and the metabolism of alcohol is complex. The body metabolizes alcohol in two steps. First, liver enzymes called alcohol dehydrogenases (ADHx) convert alcohol to a toxic chemical called acetaldehyde. Acetaldehyde is what causes many of the negative effects of drinking. Toxic to the body, it produces uncomfortable physiological responses such as headaches, facial flushing, or profuse sweating.[19]

In the second step, a group of enzymes called aldehyde dehydrogenases (ALDHs) convert acetaldehyde to a relatively harmless product called acetate, which for many people, the body easily eradicates.

But if someone has a relatively fast-acting form of ADH and slow-acting form of ALDH, then alcohol, with its euphoric effects, disappears quickly, but acetaldehyde builds up with a number of unpleasant side effects. If that person keeps drinking, he or she builds up toxic levels of acetaldehyde. For such people, their body's negative response should make them avoid alcohol.[20] However, if someone has a relatively slow-acting form of ADH and fast-acting form of ALDH, alcohol euphoria persists longer and acetaldehyde disappears quickly, so unpleasant side effects are largely avoided.[21]

Thus, certain gene-based enzymes allow some people to handle alcohol well, whereas others inherit different gene-based enzymes and don't handle alcohol as well. Obviously, before we form habits about drinking alcohol, each of us ideally needs to learn into which of these groups we fall.

Consider now an example of the role of genetics in explaining alcoholism and addiction in East Asians. Consider an Asian person who has efficient ALDH1 genes, which quickly converts alcohol acetaldehyde, but too quickly for the ALDH2 genes to handle, resulting in buildup of acetaldehyde in the body, making these Asian drinkers sick. Consider finally a specific variation of the ALDH2 gene, called ALDH2*2, that creates an enzyme that is completely inactive in metabolizing acetaldehyde to acetate. This gene is found in 60–85 percent of individuals of East Asian descent.[22]

As researcher H. J. Edenberg writes, "The *ADH1B*2* allele, which is associated with particularly rapid ethanol oxidation, has shown protective effects against alcohol dependence in a variety of populations. In East Asians, in whom the *ADH1B*2* allele is found at high frequency, *it is protective against alcoholism.*"[23]

WHY DO MOST NATIVE AMERICANS DRINK MORE THAN EAST ASIANS?

Native American ancestry is largely Siberian, so we would expect that if genes are involved, Native Americans and Siberians would have similar patterns of drinking and alcoholism. (East Asians such as Chinese and Japanese migrated from the south of Siberia and therefore have a different ancestry.) Because of the conquest of Siberia by Russia, Siberia today is populated mainly by Russians, and of its 40 million people, only about 4.5 million are the indigenous peoples related to Native Americans.

Native Americans and Alaskan Natives are five times more likely than other ethnicities in the United States to die of alcohol-related causes. Are both groups predisposed to alcoholism because of genetic differences in the way they metabolize alcohol? Possibly, but the evidence is harder to pin down than one might expect.

From the above, we know that geneticists believe that inheriting the ADH1B*2 allele creates enzymes that metabolize alcohol in ways that protect against alcoholism. Professor Cindy Ehlers of the Scripps Research Institute spent decades researching the genetic bases of alcoholism in Native Americans.

Her research led her to attack the common belief (which she calls a "myth") that "Native American Indians have a weakness for alcohol and that if they drink even small amounts of alcohol, they become uncontrolled drinkers, such that they can't handle drinking and subsequently develop alcohol addiction."[24]

Astonishingly, what Ehlers discovered is just the opposite: "Indians have a resistance to the effects of alcohol so that they can drink actually quite astronomical amounts of alcohol and not feel as intoxicated. What we've been able to show is that people who are at higher risk for developing alcoholism seem to have an inherent tolerance or a low level of response to alcohol. They need a lot more alcohol to feel intoxicated, and so they're more at risk for becoming a heavy drinker, and heavy drinking is basically the route for developing alcoholism."[25]

Overall, Ehlers believes that at least 50 percent of alcoholism, even among Native Americans, is "psychosocial," which helps explain why drinking patterns and rates of alcoholism differ among the 350 federally recognized Indian tribes.

So why do Native Americans develop such high rates of alcoholism and addiction? In a 2013 overview, Ehlers and coauthor Ian Gizer investigated the role of genetics in risk for substance dependence in Native Americans. Their conclusions are ambiguous. Although most Native Americans lack protective variants seen in other populations such as East Asians, Ehlers and Gizer found that "studies of the genes that code for alcohol-metabolizing enzymes have not revealed any risk variants specific to Native American populations."[26] Nevertheless, and somewhat strangely, they assert, "Overlap in the gene locations for substance dependence and BMI (body mass index) suggests that a common genetic substrate may exist for disorders of consumption." (In other words, the genes that make some drink make others eat too much.)

Overall, Ehlers and Gizer conclude:

> The high rates of substance dependence seen in some tribes is likely a combination of a lack of genetic protective factors (metabolizing enzyme variants) combined with genetically mediated risk factors (externalizing traits, consumption drive, and drug sensitivity or tolerance) that combine with key environmental factors (trauma exposure, early age at onset of use, and environmental hardship) to produce an elevated risk for the disorder.[27]

EVALUATION OF THE GENETICS MODEL AND NATIVE AMERICANS

This is pretty weak stuff. So Native Americans lack the protective genes that push East Asians not to drink, but that doesn't explain why Native Americans and Native Alaskans have five times the rate of alcoholic deaths as other Americans. If we compare Ehlers and Gizer's conclusions to other genetic studies of disease, the argument looks even weaker.

Consider Huntington's disease. Inheriting a gene for this terrible, progressive neurological disease is very bad. This gene is autosomal dominant, meaning each child of an affected parent has a 50 percent chance of inheriting the toxic gene. For this disease, it doesn't matter whether the victim eats only organic vegetables, takes massive dosages of Vitamin D, exercises fanatically, or does crossword puzzles all day: by the time he's on Medicare, the disease will begin, first with tremors and lastly with complete loss of memory and mental function. In other words, if someone has the gene for Huntington's, it is "fully penetrant," meaning that if the affected person lives long enough, he is sure to get Huntington's.

However, with genes for breast cancer and Alzheimer's disease, it depends on whether a person gets one copy or two copies of the relevant genes. With one copy, environmental and social factors play a role in whether or when breast cancer or Alzheimer's develops. With two copies, one is fairly certain to get breast cancer or Alzheimer's.

But nothing like any of these scenarios exists for genetics, Native Americans, and alcoholism. As Ehlers and Gizer conclude, no gene-based enzymes (or lack of them) have been discovered that predispose some Native Americans to heavy drinking.

Finally, if it's true that "Indians have a resistance to the effects of alcohol so that they can drink actually quite astronomical amounts of alcohol and not feel as intoxicated," then why do so many Indians drink so much? While it makes sense that they may damage their livers more than other people, if they need to drink more to reach the same euphoria level experienced by normal drinkers, this still doesn't explain the motive or behavior for heavy drinking. At bottom, the case for genetic causes for drinking in Native Americans remains elusive.

CRITICISMS OF THE GENETICS MODEL FROM THE SOCIAL JUSTICE MODEL

So, what other perspectives exist on Native Americans, genetics, and drinking? One powerful critique comes from Social Justice advocates. Like Ehlers, they critique the common belief that Native Americans are genetically prone—in some way or other—to alcoholism and addiction (to use slang, Native Americans "can't hold their liquor" the way whites can).

Social Justice theorists turn the table on this belief, arguing that *the belief itself* in hereditary alcoholism and addiction has been devastating to Native Americans.

Not only has this idea damaged how the public views Native Americans, but it has also been internalized by Native Americans themselves. As Roxanne Dunbar-Ortiz and Dina Gilio-Whitaker write,

> Conventional wisdom held that Native contact with alcohol led to "instant personal and cultural devastation," but a landmark study in 1969 by MacAndrew and Edgerton and subsequent studies began challenging those beliefs. In a 1971 study, anthropologist Nancy Oestreich Lurie hypothesized that drinking at some point became a way for Indians to validate and assert their Indianness in the face of negative stereotypes such as the disappearing Native. Lurie argued that Indian drinking was "the world's longest ongoing protest demonstration."[28]

While this may be an exaggeration, it does highlight what Ehlers called the "50 percent" psychosocial factors that seem to underlie heavy drinking in some tribes. Such factors also help explain why many Native American females do not drink anything like males or drink in moderation, as well as why some tribes don't allow drinking at all, and, finally, why the hundreds of different tribes in North America differ greatly in their experience with alcohol.

Social Justice theorists are essentially arguing that alcohol and opiates are instruments of dominating First Nations citizens, and for such theorists, the belief in the natural disposition of Native Americans to alcoholism may be a governing myth in such domination. Certainly, the social effect of genocide and enslavement of Native Americans has inflicted a heavy toll on them.

THE GENETICS MODEL, DESTIGMATIZING CONDITIONS, AND FATALISM

Some might argue that one important function of either genetic or neurobiological approaches to alcoholism and addiction is to destigmatize these conditions. Sometimes, the anti-moralistic desire to do so seems powerful among families of abusers and researchers, such that this fact alone justifies the model ("dopamine made me do it" or "I got drinking genes from my parents").

A similar move has been made linking homosexuality to genes. If a person's sexual orientation is not chosen or learned, but rather innate, then no one can change it and no one is responsible for their orientation.

However, the view that one is "born to do drugs" or "born to be an alcoholic" is also a powerful view, one that may make it seem inevitable that children of alcoholics or addicted people must also succumb. All things considered, let's be careful what we wish for: genetic knowledge can be both liberating and destructive.

Which brings up one problem with any deep, genetic theory of alcoholism or addiction—namely, fatalistic foreknowledge of something terrible that inevitably will happen. Recall the ancient prophecy that Oedipus, despite his attempts to avoid it, would have sex with his mother and kill his father, the king.

Fatalism is pernicious to any attempt to quit drinking or using drugs. Getting tested for Huntington's disease, when there is no treatment for it and no way of avoiding its onset, is to seek fatalistic knowledge, knowledge that might give one a "sick identity" long before any symptoms arise.

Fatalism is bleak, claiming that regardless of my personal background and my own decisions, certain events are preordained and beyond my power to change them. Calvinism and its doctrine of Predestination was fatalistic: if they were not born into the right group, nothing humans can do can get them saved. But in this Calvinist world, if one feels that one is prone to sin and, hence, not born in the right group, then what motive exists to act well and be saved? It's hopeless.

Fatalistic depression is what people fear when they hear about genetic testing for diseases that they can do nothing to prevent. Suppose someone does discover a gene variant for alcoholism or addiction, like the one for breast cancer.

The world then is divided over whether pre-symptomatic knowledge of such genetic diseases is good. If they can't do anything about it, some people prefer not to know. Others feel just the opposite: if they're going to start losing their mind at sixty, they want to know now because they're going to start to enjoy each day.

EPIGENETICS AND RISK FOR ADDICTION

Decades ago, researchers did not believe that changes in the environment could affect which genes were inherited and the makeup of genes. Several groundbreaking studies over generations, one involving starvation, showed that extreme conditions in the environment, such as lack of food or heavy use of alcohol, could affect which genes are changed and passed on to offspring.[29] Thus the new field of *epigenetics* was born—that is, the field that investigates how the expression of genes is affected by the environment of a person from the embryonic stage to late adulthood.

So far, we have discussed the Genetics model's claim that certain genes increase the risk for alcoholism and addiction. What we have not discussed is how a parent's lifelong use of drugs and alcohol might affect the risk for addiction and alcoholism of his or her future children. We are not talking here about *in utero* exposure to alcohol or opiates, but rather changes in genes carried by sperm and egg due to ongoing habits.

Epigenetics as a field is in its infancy. There are many things we don't know. Exposure before conception could affect offspring in several ways, including *reducing* the risk of addiction or alcoholism in offspring.[30]

ALL OF US

Small variations in genes also matter. Some people with AUD find that naltrexone helps them reduce their cravings, but others without the specific variation find the drug of little help.[31] Perhaps 50 percent of variations in sensitivity to pain is inheritable.[32] Pain is not studied as deeply as other medical problems because it is usually seen as a symptom, not as a continuing problem in itself, which it can be.

However, we have learned that a few humans cannot experience pain, which normally signals the brain that something is wrong. Jo Cameron, a seventy-one-year-old Scottish woman, has just such a rare genetic mutation, and scientists are studying her.[33]

Exactly how inherited genes make people vulnerable to alcoholism and addiction is hard to pinpoint, but researchers promise that "our future understanding of addictions will be enhanced by the identification of genes that have a role in altered substance-specific vulnerabilities such as variation in drug metabolism or drug receptors and a role in shared vulnerabilities such as variation in reward or stress resiliency."[34]

The Precision Medicine Initiative, commonly called "All of Us," started by NIH and Francis Collins in 2017, hopes to enroll one million Americans, map their genes and individual variations and, over decades, tease out which single nucleotide polymorphisms (SNPs) matter in causing diseases and in rates of success in responding to various treatments. This project could also reveal new insights about alcoholism and addiction. Led by the University of Alabama at Birmingham, Alabama is one of the first states to try to enroll ten thousand citizens in this project.

Consider a similar scenario involving human cloning. How much could we learn if we safely created several humans by somatic cell transfer (commonly called "cloning") from the same ancestral genotype? The hit cable show *Orphan Black* gave us some idea. Variations in how the babies from the same single ancestor were gestated and raised affected how each adult's phenotype looked. Although they all shared certain features, there were great variations among them.

Will *Orphan Black* mirror the future? How much do genes determine who we are and how much do environments? What is more important, nature or nurture? How do both interact in different ways? We don't know now, but one day we could safely originate a dozen baboon babies from the same genotype and raise them in different environments, and then we could know more. Although we shouldn't do that with humans, when cloning mammals becomes safe and efficient, we will learn a lot about genes versus environment.

In the same way, mapping genetic variations in generations of families over decades will likely give researchers a much more accurate view of genetic vulnerabilities to alcoholism and addiction. They will also discover whether receiving multiple copies of certain genes or their variations makes for stronger dispositions to alcoholism and addiction.

This may lead to the era in medicine of personalized genomics. All of Us could identify genetic variations relevant to different treatments for alcoholism and addiction.[35] For example, having the mu-opioid receptor polymorphism Asp40 may predict favorable responses to the use of naltrexone in treating alcoholic individuals.

More generally, genes have a range of expression, and that range is activated (or not) by environmental causes. A woman may inherit a risk of breast cancer, but that risk may be activated only by smoking cigarettes, using birth control pills, or being exposed to industrial chemicals. Without such exposure, her risk of developing breast cancer may be minimal.

This situation changes if she inherits not one but two copies of a gene for breast cancer. In the latter case, she may get breast cancer regardless of how she lives. If a child has two parents who are heavy drinkers and that child receives two copies of lazy genes, then that child may be much more likely than normal to become a heavy drinker. This also seems true of early-onset Alzheimer's, which can strike in the fifties, often when both parents are afflicted with the same disease.

Some people get two copies of the lazy variant of the ADH1B gene, making them doubly genetically susceptible to the pleasant effects of alcohol. If this happens (and we will one day have this kind of genetic knowledge), we will discover that some people have a very hard time refusing the pleasures of alcohol. Others might get two copies of the "efficient" genes, making them hate alcohol after a few tries.

For many diseases (alcoholism and addiction probably included), multiple genes are involved—that is, the cause of the disease is multi-genetic or polygenetic. If this is true for alcoholism and addiction, that makes prediction and treatment much harder. Given the complexities of the genetics of alcoholism in Native Americans, this personalized approach to predicting either alcoholism and addiction or treatments for them may be decades away because first we need to follow individuals and families over decades to see how patterns evolve and what environmental triggers matter most.

CRITICISMS AND EVALUATIONS OF THE GENETICS MODEL

Our review of the evidence behind a genetic basis of alcoholism in Native Americans suggests we are far from a good, tight, scientific explanation. Because so much has been written about the genetic cause of alcoholism in Native Americans, I have used such writings as a test of the Genetics model's ability to explain alcoholism.

Claims abound of researchers who adopt the Genetics model. For example, two researchers suggested that "the genetic disposition to develop alcoholism involves an initial state of central nervous system (CNS) disinhibition/ hyperexcitability" and this disposition is inherited through family lines.[36] However, these researchers offer no way to falsify or prove this hypothesis.

Researchers like the above two in genetics may write as if we already have a good model of the genetics of alcoholism and addiction, but we do not. This casts doubt on the wider applications of the Genetics model to alcoholism— for example, to Irish Americans or to any heavy drinker with alcoholic ancestors.

One hundred years ago during America's embrace of eugenics, it was fashionable to think that every human trait, vice, or disease had a genetic basis. This may be the basis for the myth that there is a single gene for alcoholism.

In the 1960s and 1970s, an opposite bias held sway, that environmental factors caused all diseases. Now the pendulum has swung to the other extreme, with scientists looking for causes of everything in genes. Is this just fashion or closer to the truth?

There is some reason to doubt the genetic explanation of alcoholism. Recall the paradigmatic example of a genetic explanation of a medical disease raised earlier in the chapter: Huntington's disease. In the case of a strong genetic connection, if you have the gene, it will be "fully penetrant" before you are sixty-five and you will likely die of it. Nothing like this exists in genetics for alcoholism.

More generally, we should ask what it means to say that "alcoholism is gene based." No pattern of familial inheritance, such as autosomal dominant or X-linked, has been established for alcoholism across generations of families. Moreover, alcoholism can skip generations, where children of alcoholics don't drink. How can a gene-based disease operate this way?

Other genetic diseases may make you crave something, such as diabetics craving sweets, so if sweets aren't around, they seek them out. If alcoholism were like that, a person who had never been exposed to alcohol would seek it out. Yet people raised in groups of teetotalers, or societies where alcohol is forbidden, do not seek alcohol. So even if it's genetic, alcoholism is a peculiar disease. Even if genes partly cause heavy drinking, it is also true that alcohol must be introduced to the person and be part of his environment.

Paul Thomas's book on alcoholism and addiction illustrates another problem with the Genetics model. He claims that "50 to 60 percent" of addiction is hereditary, and he cites his wife's physician, who "never had a drink," as the main weapon to use in fighting against such an inherited vulnerability. But in the other 99 percent of his book, he rails against "Frankenfood," lack of exercise, Big Pharma, Vitamin D deficiency, and pill-peddling physicians, but to what purpose?

If genetic vulnerabilities put some people on the bad end of the spectrum of susceptibility to alcoholism/addiction, why worry about the small stuff? Physicians in addiction medicine such as Thomas seem to contradict themselves in claiming addiction is 50–60 percent genetic and then charging clients for a dozen ways to recover from that addiction.

Finally, consider a knock-down objection to the Genetics model, especially its claim that genetic inheritance underlies the "acquired disease of the brain" model of addiction posited by neuroscience or the "medical disease" posited by Alcoholics Anonymous. If some deep, genetic structure caused some people to (1) want to drink, (2) quickly become insatiable drinkers, and (3) become unable to quit, then no one would ever quit. You can't change your genes, and if genes are making you get cancer, be bald, or be attracted to members of the same sex, then you can't change that. In one study of nearly a thousand Native Americans in four tribes, former drinkers were followed for three years. The researchers concluded, "The findings show that older adults, women, and married adults were more likely to have quit using alcohol."[37]

In a well-known study on genetics about drinking by Native Americans, although the researchers implied that most of the Native American males they interviewed were alcoholics, the researchers did note that *"many of these participants were in remission at the time of the examination"* (my emphasis).[38] Perhaps these Native American men learned, like so many other heavy drinkers, to moderate their drinking. This is compatible with the idea that having a more mature brain, or growing in maturity, helps people stop drinking.

Yes, people do stop drinking, especially in therapy. More important, and as we've emphasized, there is spontaneous remission, and some people simply become mature as adults and learn to control or even stop drinking. Not only does the Genetics model have no explanation for such cessation, but such cessation also contradicts the Genetics model.

It is conceivable that a defender of the Genetics model, when confronted with a person alleged to have inherited "drinking genes" from alcoholic parents and grandparents, might have a novel response when that person at age thirty-eight just quits drinking. Such a defender might say, "I thought you had a gene for alcoholism, but because you stopped drinking on your own, you obviously do not." But that response would be circular and make the theory non-falsifiable.

Champions of the Coping model also chime in here, arguing that it's always hard to distinguish between genes causing alcoholism in families and learned ways of coping with depression and stress in the same families.

Consider again Ernie Crowfeather. Does the Genetics model help explain his drinking? By all accounts, he was handsome and charming. Physicians and relatives repeatedly tried to save him, even violating protocols to do so. Why did someone with everything to live for keep drinking, knowing it was harming his failed kidneys? Are genes the only, or even best, explanation here? What about depression? Maybe antidepressants would have helped. Maybe his crisis was personal and existential, in which case a good counselor may have helped. Or was he simply immature and made a series of increasingly bad decisions, for which he was ultimately responsible? In the final analysis, Ernie's tragic death remains a mystery.

By contrast, consider the "lethal" party described at the beginning of this chapter by famous Native American writer Sherman Alexie, who grew up in eastern Washington. The fights at that party and the dangerous, drunken antics among Indians, especially among his father and his friends, so scared his mother that the next morning she fled in a car with her children to her hometown, hoping to never return to the reservation. With no resources, she had to return with her children, but a day later, after cleaning the house, "she woke us, her children, and promised us that she would stop drinking booze that very second and would never drink again. . . . She was sober for the rest of her life."[39]

CONCLUSIONS

A comprehensive review of genes and addictions in 2009 concluded that understanding the genetic expression of alcoholism and addictions is at present "very limited."[40]

If a genetic basis for alcoholism and addiction exists, it should fulfill at least one of two major conditions: first, most of those with the genes who are exposed to alcohol or opiates should develop substance abuse; second, every alcoholic or addicted person should have inherited, on investigation, the relevant genes. Yet, despite frequent claims by genetic researchers and others that genes account for at least half the dispositions to drink and use drugs, no study seems to have met either condition.[41]

Moreover, a flip side exists to the problem of fatalism. If thinking your drinking or injecting is caused by your genes is one kind of problem, then thinking it is caused *only* by the genes is another. Those who lack the "alcoholism genes" or the "addiction genes" may feel immune from ever having serious problems from drinking or using opiates.

Summary of the Genetics Model

Underlying cause: Dispositions to alcoholism and addiction have a biological basis in inherited genes. Whether and how genes are expressed depends on complex, epigenetic factors such as repeated exposure to addictive substances and secondary gains from using such substances. But evidence shows that alcoholism and addiction run in certain families and ethnic groups, almost never in other families and other ethnic groups.

Treatment: The focus should be on research to understand how to prevent inherited tendencies from being expressed in toxic ways. If genes for alcoholism and addiction are identified, some parents using assisted reproduction might want to "de-select" embryos of babies containing those genes in favor of embryos without those genes.

Other models: Seeing addiction only as a matter of one person or one family goes only so far in explaining why addiction runs so rampant in some families and ethnic groups. If addiction has even a partial basis in genes, that is important to know, both for families and for affected individuals.

Responsibility: People are not responsible for the genes they inherit or the dispositions those genes give them. Genetics, with its core in deep biology, comes closest to fatalism, especially if genes for addiction and alcoholism are discovered and if having two copies of those genes doubles chances of alcoholism or addiction. Although it sounds gimmicky, according to this view, people suffering from alcoholism and addiction can almost truthfully say, "My genes make me do it."

Family matters: If genes for alcoholism or addiction are discovered, prospective parents should consider using assisted reproduction and testing embryos for these genes, with a plan of only implanting unaffected embryos.

BAD WAYS OF COPING

> You don't wake up one morning and decide to be a drug addict. It takes at least three months' shooting twice a day to get any habit at all. . . . I think it not exaggeration at all to say it takes about a year and several hundred injections to make an addict.
>
> —William S. Burroughs, *Junky*

O n the day-to-day basis of helping addicted individuals and problem drinkers function in our society, no one lives more on the front lines than clinical psychologists, social workers, psychiatrists, and counselors. It is this group that requires urgent, practical advice about how to help. It is this group that most immediately knows what works. It is also this group's members who personally experience the fatalities caused by our opioid epidemic and rampant alcoholism.

So we should not be surprised if members of this group lack interest in grand theories but instead expect (and offer) practical advice about living without drugs or alcohol.

BACKGROUND

When the director of the National Institute on Drug Abuse, Nora Volkow, MD, and her colleagues wrote an essay in 2016 in the *New England Journal of Medicine* that called addiction a "disease of the brain,"[1] their view did not go unchallenged. Two years later, Marc Lewis, a professor of psychology at the University of Toronto and Radboud University in the Netherlands, rebutted this view in the same journal in his essay titled "Brain Change in Addiction as Learning, Not Disease."[2]

In his essay, Lewis defended what we shall call the Coping model of addiction, which sees alcoholism or addiction as learned ways of coping with bad things in life, such as stress, physical injury, or lack of meaning. This model is "external" because it focuses on actions and behavior, rather than something "internal" such as genes or neural circuits.

A neuroscientist, Lewis was himself in recovery from addiction, a story he recounts in *The Biology of Desire: Why Addiction Is Not a Disease*.[3] In his essay, Lewis notes that the disease model is the most prevalent model of addiction in the Western world.

How did this come about? Lewis's answer is that "twelve-step thinking" converged with residential treatment models in the latter half of the twentieth century at the same time that an explosion of neuroimaging technologies began in the 1990s. A convergence of professionals and community advocates from both groups passionately promoted the disease model to the detriment of traditional models such as the Coping model.

Although Professor Lewis agrees that the disease model is useful in some contexts, especially for reducing moral stigma and for securing funding for research in medical labs, its narrow focus diverts attention (and research funding) from models that emphasize the social and environmental causes of addiction.

In other words, when the brain-disease model of addiction allied with AA/NA's disease model, the two crowded out the Coping model, which claimed that addiction stemmed from learned social roles and habit-forming behavior. Subsequently, in treating and explaining addiction, when pharmacologically oriented psychiatrists replaced clinical psychologists and medical sociologists, important aspects of the addict's life dropped out from discussions of treatment.

Like Lewis, science writer Maia Szalavitz believes that neuroscientists have hijacked funding for research in addiction medicine. Szalavitz is the most important living science writer who specializes in reporting about addiction. A recovering addict herself, she was raised as a gifted child and got a scholarship to an Ivy League university.[4] Nevertheless, at age twenty-three she found herself injecting heroin and cocaine up to forty times a day. She overcame her addiction and then started a journey to understand why she succeeded and why others did not.

Sally Satel, a practicing psychiatrist, agrees that the Neuroscience model offers little day-to-day help for addiction doctors trying to help patients. She argues in *Brainwashed: The Seductive Appeal of Neuroscience* that "knowledge of the neural mechanisms underlying addiction typically has less relevance to the treatment of drug addiction than the psychological and social causes."[5]

In her book, Szalavitz agrees, arguing that our understanding of addiction is trapped in unfounded ideas, such as the claim by neuroscientists that addiction is only a disease of the brain. Three years later, she sounded the alarm in the *New York Times* that physicians had cut back so much in prescribing opiates for pain relief that some patients were suicidal or in unremitting pain.[6]

Szalavitz strongly believes that addictions are disorders of learning. She argues that understanding them this way best serves people struggling to recover, best guides public policy about treating and preventing addiction, and best agrees with the facts.

She claims something that surprises some. For her, addictive behaviors fall on a spectrum of learning disorders comparable to autism. For her, the user's brain isn't broken, but it developed in an aberrant way, comparable to the brains of people with attention deficit hyperactivity disorder (ADHD) or autism spectrum disorder. In her words, "Like ADHD or autism, addiction is what you might call a wiring difference, not necessarily a destruction of tissue."[7]

More globally, she gives evidence that addictive behaviors are quasi-normal responses to trauma, abuse, poverty, and crisis. For most addicts, she sensibly argues, no single treatment works for all. Rather, a confluence of history, family, and culture is what engenders both addiction and the recovery.

Neuroscience and genetics tend to leave out of the discussion how race, class, gender, and context affect human behavior. Each adult makes decisions in a culture that embraces or eschews ritualistic consumption of alcohol; each adult makes decisions having grown up watching his parents and relatives consume alcohol rarely, moderately, or excessively; each adult makes decisions either as a member of a privileged class—knowing that if he makes mistakes, he has family and money to brace him—or knowing that, being from a lower economic class, he is likely to make the same mistakes as his peers.

In terms of likelihood of recovery, it seems obvious that people with a strong sense of familial or ethnic identity, who have a sense of self and purpose in life, are far better able to successfully cope with alcohol and opiates, even if they might be genetically disposed. Equally important, when they become dependent on alcohol or opiates, people in these circumstances are far more likely to mature out and learn to cope with normal life without drugs or alcohol.

Cognitive-behavioral models of therapy fall under the Coping model. Therapists help clients with substance abuse problems and focus on why they need alcohol or opioids to have satisfying relationships or why they avoid such relationships by retreating into alcohol or narcotics. Cognitive-behavioral psychotherapy, most often practiced by clinical psychologists and other counselors, uses the power of self-analysis and insight to change patterns of destructive behavior.

Szalavitz fiercely attacks the dominant view of addiction as a progressive disease of the brain. Her first book, *Help at Any Cost*, exposed the tough-love model that dominated rehab centers for troubled teens.[8] These programs espoused harsh measures and strict enforcement of rules to get people to end their self-destructive ways. Szalavitz argues that the Coping model provides a better way of understanding how people get addicted: "In both autism and addictions, for example, repetitive coping behaviors frequently are misinterpreted as the source of the problem, rather than being seen as attempts at solutions."[9] She disputes the claim of other models that addiction results from exposure to a drug by a person with a certain kind of inherited personality or brain dysfunction. Instead, she sees addiction as a learned relationship between exposure to drugs and a person's overall dispositions, which in turn are created by her environment, her family, and her emotional needs.

Szalavitz repeatedly emphasizes that just removing drugs from repeat users, without teaching those users how to cope with life's problems, is "like trying to ban compulsive hand washing by banning one soap after another."[10]

For Coping model theorists, maturity matters in escaping addiction. They emphasize that addiction is much less common in people who first try drugs over the age of twenty-five and that most users quit by the time they reach their mid-thirties. One study reports that the prefrontal cortex of the brain regulates decision-making, social behavior, and good judgment. This area of the brain is not fully developed until about twenty-five years of age (and generally females mature faster than males).[11] Thus, older people are able to cope with problems without using drugs.

Like Marc Lewis, Szalavitz describes how the Coping model explains why good employment and the support of family matter so much in who recovers and who does not—factors that the Genetics and Neuroscience models remain silent about. Part of this is surely correct because drinking or using drugs doesn't occur in a vacuum. Think of a user as the center of vortex of forces acting to move the person in different directions, some toward safety, some toward danger. Each individual will deal with these forces differently. When people have good family connections and role models assuring him of eventual success and happiness, dependency on drugs or alcohol is less likely.

The Coping model also explains why punishment doesn't work. What people learn when they are punished for using drugs is to avoid punishment, not to stop using drugs. Thus, criminalization of alcoholism and addiction, as well as tough love and interventionist models popular in NA/AA groups, all miss the point. For Szalawitz, understanding addiction as a learning disorder first means to understand "that it is actually defined by resistance to punishment."[12]

COPING WITHOUT DRUGS OR ALCOHOL WITH NEW PARTNERS AND FRIENDS

To take another example from Coping model therapists, it is well known that addicted people often live in pairs, and when one member of the pair tries to go clean without the other also doing so, it may break up the relationship. By contrast, if a heavy drinker switches to a teetotalist (completely abstinent) partner, it is much easier for him to stay in permanent recovery. In rehab groups, former addicts and alcoholics are advised that they must find new friends and cannot go back to hanging out with those with whom they used to get high.

Who we live with matters, affecting how we fail or flourish. For example, after a decade of abuse, philosopher Owen Flanagan cites his family as the only reason he kicked methamphetamines and alcohol.[13] In one case known to the author, a midlife alcoholic who had been in several month-long, expensive, residential treatment programs stopped using only when, after driving with her grandchildren while drunk, she was barred from ever seeing them again unless she completely stopped drinking. In both cases, the power of families taking a stance changed bad behavior and helped someone recover. The Neuroscience model has no explanation for how such occurrences work.

One crucial question is whether a person can stop drinking or using when he or she is in a long-term relationship in which drinking or using figures prominently. Many people in recovery would answer "no" and attest to the power of being around new friends who do not drink or use. Certainly, if drinking is a central focus of someone's life and remains the focus of that person's partner, finding a new partner who is not drinking will be a major help in quitting. Some counselors in addiction therapy claim it is necessary for recovery.

A related question is whether a person can stop drinking or using when he or she hangs around with the same friends or associates. Again, if drinking or using is a central focus of the friends, a person trying to quit cannot be around them as before. As the work of social psychologist Stanley Milgram taught us about obedience to authority, the social context of our actions can be very powerful in determining how we act, and only fools ignore that context.[14]

THE COPING MODEL AND DEFINITIONS OF ADDICTION

If we conceptualize alcoholism or addiction as a somewhat mysterious, hidden, biological disease—whether genetic, chemical, or neurological—then treatments must repair damaged genes, chemical imbalances, or broken brains. However, if heavy drinking every day is merely a learned behavior, then drinkers may be able to quickly learn more functional ways of handling alcohol.

Definitions are important, especially for drinkers and how they see themselves. Recall the discussion in the chapter on Alcoholics Anonymous about suggestibility and labels. A big difference exists between "I have a brain disease" and "I drink in stupid ways."

Consider two narratives about famous surgeon William Halsted, the chief of surgery at Johns Hopkins Hospital in Baltimore. The first comes from AA/NA and biological-genetic perspectives that see Halsted as suffering from the disease of addiction to cocaine. For critics, Halsted's superiors let him get away with secret, daily usage at his home behind locked doors and the occasional binges while away in North Carolina or Europe. He never admitted his problem, never faced his addiction, and never became the ideal mentor to his surgical residents.

An alternative narrative is this: Like many physicians of his day, Halsted in his twenties had easy access to cocaine, which was first seen as a non-addicting substitute for heroin (Halsted's contemporary, Sigmund Freud, argued this way for years). By the time cocaine's addictive potential was widely known, physicians such as Halsted had become dependent. By then in his mid-thirties and head of surgery at Hopkins, Halsted knew that his use of cocaine could be his downfall (he had been caught once and forced into residential rehab, which almost derailed his career). He thus allowed himself to use cocaine only when alone, either in his room or away on travels. He attended his patients each morning and afternoon. And because he knew he would be high, he instituted a system where his surgical residents knew they could not contact him after 4:00 p.m. Halsted gave them amazing authority and independence—the same with his junior surgeons on faculty. This demanding system of the surgical residency program at Hopkins soon became the model for the entire country, even the world. And it all came about because of one brilliant surgeon's method of coping with his dependence on cocaine.

The two narratives differ substantially in how they view essentially the same pattern of behavior. One makes Halsted into a Dr. Jekyll and Mr. Hyde tale, with Mr. Hyde ravaged by a terrible disease. The other makes Halsted the hero of his own story, a surgeon who triumphed over a dependency that brought down many others addicted to cocaine during his time.

Two similar, contrasting narratives could be told about William Wilberforce, the parliamentarian who led Britain's battle to end the slave trade and who lived addicted to opium for forty-five years.[15] Wilberforce's biographers tend to assume that because he was a morally good person, he was not really addicted, or, if he was really addicted, he was not really a good person. It seems hard for any biographer to accept that he could have been a good person and lived a normal life while still struggling with opium.

In some cities, physicians who specialize in addiction medicine run groups on weeknights for addicted dentists, nurses, anesthesiologists, surgeons, and others.[16] Each night, each person provides a urine sample and pays $100 in cash (for various reasons, no insurance is billed).

Each person has been identified as an impaired physician, dentist, teacher, or nurse. Each has made a deal with a hospital, practice, or licensing board to enter weekly treatment in this way and continue employment. By doing so, each maintains the income that pays for mortgages, college tuition, and weekly expenses, as well as a sense of purpose in working as a professional. So long as each shows up each week, pays, and tests clean, each can continue working.

Is this such a bad deal? From the point of view of most models, the people in these groups are just treading water, not really swimming toward any goal. Some may even be on substitution or maintenance drugs. But Harm Reduction certainly approves, and all participants in these groups are learning to function at work without using alcohol or drugs, so the Coping model highly approves.

The Coping model is usually unhappy with the many models in psychology, counseling, and rehab that insist on delving into a substance abuser's childhood and family relations. One of the crucial assumptions of many therapy groups for treating alcoholism or addiction is that using drugs or heavy drinking is a symptom of much deeper personal problems, and, as such, treatment of alcoholism or addiction must focus on solving those problems. Hence the dominant assumption in our culture that treating the alcoholism and addiction must involve twelve steps, being in a group and honestly discussing one's faults, and, ideally, being in one-on-one psychotherapy with a therapist who specializes in treating these problems.

A corollary of this assumption is that there is something deeply wrong with addicted people or heavy drinkers. They are escaping from life's problems, frustrations at work, an unhappy marriage, or divorcing parents. A second corollary is that if the addicted person becomes more fulfilled, happy at work, and involved in a good marriage or relationship, his use of drugs or alcohol will diminish or stop.

Jack Trimpey is a social worker who worked for decades with alcoholic patients and is a recovering heavy drinker. Advocating the Harm Reduction model, he has consistently attacked the rehab industry and its claim that heavy drinking or using drugs is a disease. In nicely cutting to the chase, he accepts that reduction of physical craving may require drug substitutes, but he advocates a far simpler idea than the mental reformation advocated by Buddhists or deep-self therapists:

> Addiction to alcohol or drugs is a devotion to pleasure produced by the substance, an ineffable self-indulgence that ultimately becomes a condition of chemically enhanced stupidity. Pleasure seeking, sometimes called "hedonism," is a natural human trait signifying health. Addiction, however, goes further than hedonism . . . into "hyperhedonism," a surpassing devotion to the specific pleasure given by certain substances. Because there is no disease, there is no "treatment" and no "cure" in the medical sense of these words.[17]

Trimpey argues that we should forget about all the deep reasons for someone's use of drugs or drinking and just focus on getting them off the pleasure-seeking habits that they've grown into. Although he disagrees with Harm Reduction's acceptance of moderate usage, he otherwise goes beyond the Coping model in rejecting the need for drinkers to focus on family relationships or early childhood. Instead of these deep, potentially unsolvable problems, let's just focus on the drinking or drugs!

In some ways, Trimpey's model accepts the idea that people can mature and abandon their rash, youthful, sensation-seeking ways. And if immaturity was the basic problem before, then nothing "deeper" needs to be cured for someone to learn to control their usage. It's also refreshing in ceasing to look for deeper causes of drug usage: even for Sigmund Freud, sometimes a cigar is just a cigar.

As a veteran social worker with limited resources treating clients who themselves often cannot get formal treatment, social worker Trimpey's practical model makes sense for his clients. It's as if Trimpey is saying, "Hey, we may not be able to fix your marriage, but we can fix your drinking (which—by the way—probably isn't helping your marriage). And, hey, we may not be able to fix your toxic relationship with your abusive father, but we can fix your habit of drinking whenever you think about him. And, hey, as a fifty-five-year-old adult, we may not be able to find your dream job, but we can fix your drinking, which surely isn't helping you get your dream job (and doing so may keep you from getting fired)." And to all that, Harm Reductionists say, "Amen." Nor do they accept, as we will see in discussing Social Justice, that we must wait for the perfect society before we can help addicted people.

It goes without saying that Harm Reductionists don't accept the concept of "dry drunk syndrome," newly articulated in 1970 as part of AA's twelve-step program and defined as a condition where individuals stop drinking but do not deal with the deeper personal and social issues that led them to become abusive drinkers.[18]

In some ways, the idea of dry drunk syndrome—more technically called Post-Acute Withdrawal Syndrome (PAWS)—is analogous to cleaning a dirty rug: you can vacuum the dirt of the top layers, but to really get it like new, you need deep cleaning. For counselors who push this concept, to be fully recovered, you need to not only stop drinking but also stop all the activities associated with your drinking.[19]

But consider a sixty-year-old marathon runner who once bought into the myth that as long as he could run marathons, he couldn't be an alcoholic. By the time he finally conquered his drinking, he had been divorced and become estranged from his adult children. He also engaged in group runs on Wednesday evenings and Sunday afternoons with a local running club, after which everyone would drink from a keg.

Sober, he still runs marathons, and sometimes he joins the running club on Wednesdays or Sundays, but he no longer joins them afterward to drink from the keg. Sometimes he even gets a buzz thinking about the times when he did drink from the keg, but he never succumbs. But he still likes to run with his old running buddies.

Is he a "dry drunk"? Even if he doesn't drink? What would count as being over this condition? Does he need to get remarried, stop running with his old group, and rebond with his children, just to feel he's out of the woods? Is he courting grave danger by engaging in previous behavior leading to heavy drinking? Some counselors would say so.

In the worst case the author ever heard, a forty-year-old woman had been diagnosed with alcoholism in her mid-twenties. She entered counseling and quit drinking by the time she was thirty. Twenty years later, at fifty, she was still in counseling for "alcoholism," although she hadn't had a drink in two decades. Her counselor had convinced her that until she solved *all* her problems, the Beast could reappear any day.

CRITICISM BY OTHER MODELS OF THE COPING MODEL

As the Coping model is the first "outside-the-body" model of addiction we've discussed, it should be clear that the "inside-the-body" models won't think it correct. Thus, both the Neuroscience and the Genetics models will tend to think it superficial, using "talk therapy" when the reality is found in neurons, synapses, and genes.

Advocates of disease models doubt any treatment that accepts moderate drinking/usage rather than complete abstinence. Some treatments promise to help you moderate or control drinking or using, they would say, but it is your Beast that leads you onto that path.[20] Believing that "the Beast" is always lurking like a predator, champions of the disease model abhor opening any door.

The Coping model will always be attacked from AA/NA as too soft and for tolerating tapered usage. As the Coping model denies almost everything in AA/NA, so AA/NA must see almost every tenet of the Coping model as letting addicted people off too easily. This is especially true with drug crimes, where AA frequently sees prison as a version of hitting bottom, whereas the Coping model thinks prison almost always worsens addiction and alcoholism.

Thus, the Coping model can be attacked from all directions, both from those seeing addiction as inside the body (Genetics and Neuroscience) and by AA/NA. And, as we shall see, it can also be attacked "from above," by Social Justice model theorists, as not getting a big enough handle on an epidemic problem. Kantians are probably the most sympathetic to the Coping model, so long as the Coping model doesn't absolve people of responsibility for their actions.

CONCLUSIONS

The Coping model adds two things lacking in the AA/NA model and Neuroscience model: first, the personal-social context of substance abuse, and second, evidence-based evaluations of different routes to recovery.

The strongest theme of the Coping model is that to be drug free, we don't need to solve all the problems of an addicted person. Ditto for alcohol dependency. Rather than conceptualize the problem as an enemy, a hidden disease, think of it as learned behavior, the wrong behavior for having fun or dealing with stress. Everyone can learn new skills, and that's a much more hopeful, practical approach than waiting for scientists to discover the hidden neural pathways of addiction, the genetic dispositions, or how to construct the perfect, drug-free society.

None of this is to say that learning to cope with life's problems is easy; people dependent on alcohol or opiates are likely to have some big problems.

Summary of the Coping Model

Underlying cause: Alcoholism and addiction are learned behaviors, which can be unlearned, mainly as reactions to trauma, boredom, stress, depression, and abuse.

Treatment: Focus on understanding past maladaptive behaviors and how better coping behaviors can be learned. Treatment should not only treat the individual's brain or his past behavior but also be located within his relationships to a partner, parents, siblings, friends, and coworkers.

Other models: Seeing addiction as a biological disease doesn't work for many users; disease models and the AA/NA typically see alcoholism/addiction as a problem of the individual, ignoring codependent partners and families. These models don't explain why most users stop on their own.

Responsibility: Users can learn to cope with life's ills without alcohol or narcotics; users can learn to take responsibility for their actions that previously harmed others and themselves.

Family matters: There is rarely a lone individual who drinks or uses opiates without a sibling, partner, or parent nearby. Sometimes that person is codependent and enables the substance abuser. For successful recovery, all parties need help the affected relative. Relatives need to learn to overcome denial, manipulation, and dishonesty by their loved one. Finally, it is false that change can only happen by a deep, inner decision by the affected relative. In some cases, pressure from family for change is the most powerful tool available for recovery.

BEYOND THE
INDIVIDUAL

Robin Williams, after becoming addicted to cocaine and
alcohol, had kicked both and lived sober for years until one
day in Skagway, Alaska, in a long interlude between filming
scenes for an upcoming movie, he began serious drinking
again: "My film career was not going well. One day I walked
into a store and saw a little bottle of Jack Daniel's. And that
voice—I call it the lower power—goes, 'Hey. Just a taste.
Just one.' I drank it, and there was a brief moment of 'Oh,
I'm okay!' "

—Dave Itzkoff, *Robin*[1]

Vancouver today features many rich communities such as Coal Harbor,
where dozens of new, expensive, high-rise condominiums overlook a
marina of yachts and, across the bay, beautiful, snow-capped mountains.
Much of this spectacular city indicates wealth and privilege.

Hidden across town a few miles on its east side is North America's first safe-
injection facility, named Insite. Following Hastings Street from west to east,
seedy buildings begin to appear, as well as the homeless—some living under
cardboard boxes on sidewalks, others rummaging through waste baskets for
deposits on cans and bottles. Ten blocks farther east, nearing Insite itself,
addicted people swarm the streets, huddled under blankets and tarps on concrete sidewalks. Down alleyways nearby, others haggle, exchanging things.
Ravaged street people push other wild-looking people in wheelchairs; ampu-
tees hobble on crutches; open-air markets flourish on every corner, where loud
arguments can be heard. This human sea rumbles with yells, screams, and
often an approaching siren.

This is the epicenter of opiate addiction in Vancouver, where Insite tries to prevent a repeat of the three thousand fatal overdoses that occurred here between 2015 and 2017. And these people have many problems, including mental illness, hepatitis, HIV, infections, and overdoses from taking fentanyl instead of heroin.

Apart from the visibly addicted people on these streets, thousands of other addicted people live inside somewhere, and hundreds of thousands of others live around Vancouver in British Columbia.

They contrast starkly with the rich people in western Vancouver. How did these street people get addicted in this rich city? Unlike Philadelphia's Kensington neighborhood, most addicted people in Vancouver are white. How did this beautiful city, with its hundreds of new, luxury condos, help create so many addicted people? How did it become a bastion of unequal life prospects?

Vancouver and Kensington are not alone. In São Paulo, Brazil, *paco* addicts live on similar streets.[2] In Tehran, they live under bridges, addicted to cheap heroin from neighboring Afghanistan. Afghanistan itself contains hundreds of thousands of opium addicts. Russia has millions of addicted IV-drug users. Nor should we leave out Great Britain, where three million citizens live on addictive drugs.

To such questions, the Social Justice model seeks answers, especially to its master question: How does the structure of one society encourage addiction and alcoholism, while the structure of another discourages it?

A MODEL OF SOCIAL JUSTICE FOR ADDICTION

The models previously discussed in this book focused on the addicted person: his genes, his coping mechanisms, his brain, his choices, and how to help him. None of them addressed Vancouver's problem and how it came about. Surely, champions of the Social Justice model argue, we can't just focus on addicted individuals and leave it at that, can we? Something profound happened in Vancouver and in Kensington. Shouldn't we try to understand what happened and why? Shouldn't there be some occasions where we take a larger view of addiction and widespread binge drinking?

To understand the Social Justice model's perspective on addiction, consider that many North Americans admit to being addicted to something: alcohol, narcotics, tobacco, sex, video games, gambling, pornography, shopping, social media, the internet, or junk food. North of the Rio Grande, we seem to be a continent of self-described addicts.

How did we get here? For social justice theorists, Big Pharma, Big Tobacco, and Big Alcohol push us into addiction. Soon Big Cannabis will make its own push (see chapter 11). Others pushing us into addiction are Big Agribusiness (processed, overly sugared foods), Big Gambling (from casinos to state lotteries to newly legalized betting on sports), and every little convenience store that sells alcohol, lottery scratch-tickets, Juul, and quick food. "Drug store" chains long ago stopped selling only drugs, as some countries require them to do, and started selling tobacco, alcohol, and lots of candy.

Social justice theorists ask us to look at how our addictions profit huge international companies. Such companies use every tool of social science to market their goods and, increasingly, to make our daily life dependent on buying such goods.

JOHN RAWLS AND HIS THEORY OF JUSTICE

One of the greatest theorists of social justice of our times was Harvard philosopher John Rawls. His *Theory of Justice* famously lays out a philosophical framework for judging whether a society is just.[3] Rawls once called his basic idea *justice as fairness*. He argued that justice applies to the basic structure of society. Health care is part of that structure.

According to Rawls, two main principles of justice exist. But how do we choose such principles or know about them? Rawls asks us to imagine a social contract where citizens choose under a *veil of ignorance* about their age, race, religion, sex, health, wealth, abilities, and talents, so they cannot bias their choices by considering their arbitrary personal characteristics. Under these conditions, Rawls believes that rational people would first choose those structures that give people *maximal equal liberty*. This is his first principle of justice: design the basic structures of a just society to give citizens maximal equal liberty.

Rawls recognized that the world is naturally unfair: some people are born into rich families, some into poor ones; some are born healthy, others with spina bifida. Government can either worsen such inequalities or lessen them. For Rawls, just governments should reduce natural inequality while preserving equal liberty. How can we do this? Answer: Some liberty can be sacrificed to achieve greater equality. When? For Rawls, inequality is justifiable when it works to the advantage of those who are worst off. We would choose this under the veil of ignorance because, when it lifts, we might be that worst-off person. So, Rawls appeals to the natural self-interest of people while forcing them to choose through the lens of (what is essentially) the Golden Rule.

Rawls's second principle of justice is something called the *difference principle*. Its name comes from when a just society allows a subsystem to differ from equal liberty (also called "fair equality of opportunity"). This principle comes into play when such a difference benefits the least well-off group while still preserving the basic priority of equal liberty.

So, physicians can make more money so long as everyone has (1) an equal opportunity to become a physician and (2) the unequal, great income of physicians motivates people to a life in medicine of serving others, especially the poorest, sickest patients.

How does such a Rawlsian view apply to addiction and alcoholism?

According to Rawls's difference principle, our present economic structure is just only if the poor are better off under it than under another system. In our present, unequal society, that is not the case.

Underlying Rawls's approach to justice is the ability to imagine ourselves as the worst-off members of the society—to see ourselves as addicted, hurt, poor, and uninsured; to imagine how bad it would be to have a serious addiction and how much worse it would be to have no way to get the care we need.

Second, Rawlsian justice asks whether the basic structure of our society is arranged to allow corporations to create addicted people and profit from them or to discourage such addictions.

Social Justice theorists urge everyone to appreciate how Oxycontin lacked the stigma of heroin and cocaine. Especially when taken after an accident, taking Oxycontin did not seem like a big deal.

For Social Justice theorists, something unique occurred in North America around 2000 that did not occur elsewhere. Systems of financial reimbursement allowed some drug companies and their employees to become quick millionaires by pushing opiates on vulnerable people.

One bad thing piggy-backed on another: (1) Oxycontin was already more powerful than previous drugs and (2) Purdue Pharma and Insys aggressively oversold it, causing millions of vulnerable people to become addicted. Coping strategies for alcohol and marijuana that worked for parents and grandparents no longer worked for the newly addicted because their dependency levels were off the charts.

Take West Virginia. Suddenly, fatal overdoses started there, as well as along the Ohio River. Those aged eighteen to thirty-five, with immature brains (and hence immature lifestyles), were easy targets. Something evil had crept into these areas.

Is there any doubt that something at the foundations of American society went wrong? Something that did not occur in Germany, France, or Russia? Although Americans like to think we have the best society in the world, in this particular aspect, was it the worst? Did loopholes in regulation of prescribing a new drug destroy the lives of millions of people and condemn their families to untold misery?

HISTORY, THE LEAST WELL OFF, AND DRUGS

Before we consider addicted people in modern North America, consider how past societies in China, North America, and Mexico dealt with alcohol and drugs and their most vulnerable populations. "Vulnerable" is used here because of its meaning in research ethics, where it connotes marginalized populations.

Historically, as we saw in our discussion in chapter 8 of the Genetics model and the First Peoples, opiates and alcohol have often been used by the wealth-owning elite to control and exploit the masses and, at the same time, to blame them for their inherent weakness of will in succumbing to these vices.

China and the Opium Wars

For almost two thousand years, the Middle Kingdom reigned as a world power and controlled its own destiny. According to one historian of economics, China in 1820 had the largest economy in the world.[4] Then Europeans began fierce fights over who would control this economy.

Opium has been used for relief of pain perhaps for as long as ten thousand years, but since it was first discovered, it has also caused addiction.[5] During the eighteenth and nineteenth centuries, Europeans learned to control Chinese workers with opium.

In essence, British officials and merchants learned that they could control Chinese workers by smuggling opium grown in Afghanistan and India into China, starting in 1787 with four thousand chests a year and growing to thirty thousand chests by 1833. Opium was later used to control low-paid "coolies" working in slave-like conditions while constructing American railroads.

China struggled with limiting opium's damage during the nineteenth century, when it fought the British Empire during the Opium Wars. When twelve million Chinese people had become addicted, especially workers in port cities, the Chinese emperor decided to resist, destroying twenty thousand chests of opium at one point and banning British ships from disembarking their cargoes.

The emperor's action led to the First Opium War, where the British Royal Navy used its guns and troops to defeat Chinese troops and ensure that British merchants could continue to supply opium to Chinese workers. The Second Opium War between 1856 and 1860 secured Britain's rights over trade in China and secured Britain's and America's right to hire cheap Chinese labor in their territories.

Looking back, social justice theorists might not blame modern Chinese for distrusting the benevolence of the English-speaking world. It is also ironic that today the tables have turned, and China makes some of the fentanyl sold to addicted North Americans and Europeans.

Mexico and North America

Social Justice theorists think that America's War on Drugs has been a failure not only for North America but especially for Mexico, Central America, and South America. Beyond putting millions of black and brown Americans behind bars for minor drug offenses, the War on Drugs has fueled devastating drug wars in Mexico, where more than a quarter million Mexicans have been killed and another forty thousand have disappeared.[6]

Citing the futility of building a wall to stop the flow of drugs, columnist George Will notes that 30 million Americans pay $150 billion for drugs smuggled from Mexico. Such drugs enter the United States inside the 4,500 trucks that each day enter three legal, huge plazas that allow entry along the border.[7] Will cites Don Winslow's best-selling trilogy, which describes the last decades of our War on Drugs and its horrible legacy of death and corruption in Mexico.[8]

Have things gotten better or worse in North America after forty years of the War on Drugs? In 1979, a milligram of pure heroin cost $9, but today it costs only 25 cents. Today, prisons contain thirty times more drug users than forty years ago.

Yet even when we lock up drug dealers, someone always takes their place. Today's dealers use cell phones, texting, social media, and child runners to deliver goods as fast as home-delivered pizza. And fentanyl will not be the last highly potent synthetic opiate to exceed the high of heroin, just the first, as drug labs tweak new, synthetic opioids.

INCREASING STRUCTURAL INEQUALITY IN AMERICA AND THE WORLD

After the recession of 2007–2009, while Americans consumed more alcohol and opiates, inequality increased. For Social Justice model theorists, part of the truth about our alcoholism and addiction stems from this growing economic inequality.

Social Justice theorists believe that between 1990 and 2020, American society became more unequal in ownership of wealth.[9] During this time, free trade, globalization, and high tech changed our lives. Highly intelligent, tech-savvy people moved to big cities on both coasts or immigrated to North America, working for Facebook, Microsoft, Google, Amazon, and Verizon, while manufacturing jobs moved to developing countries such as China and Mexico with low-paid workers. As a result, a few talented, lucky people became billionaires, such as hedge fund billionaire Ken Griffin, who in 2019 paid a whopping $238 million for a penthouse in Manhattan, the largest amount ever paid for a residence there.

These developments created a semi-permanent underclass in North America, leaving many towns in rural parts of America, largely composed of people over fifty, with fewer jobs in manufacturing, the traditional job that led to middle-class security for people without college degrees. The pattern repeated in France, where the Yellow Vests in 2019 protested the growing structural inequality that had hit them hard.

At the same time, millions of students in college took on high levels of debt—debt that could never be forgiven through bankruptcy and that shackled future earnings. Millennials, those born between 1980 and 2000, were often hard hit. Because of debt from college and lack of well-paying jobs, they frequently put off marriage and buying a house. Structural inequality for them may be lifelong.

West Virginia, Inequality, and Addiction

Consider West Virginia, which had one of the highest rates of addiction in America. Between 2016 and 2017, it also had the highest rate of overdose fatalities, nearly fifty deaths per 100,000 citizens, compared to nine for Alabama and three for Nebraska.[10]

For a hundred years before, working in coal mines and steel plants allowed West Virginians to enjoy a good life, even those who only completed ninth grade. As mines and plants closed, similar jobs did not replace them, leading to unemployment and a class of resentful, largely white, citizens.

One of the easiest ways to survive without having a job was to get disability payments, which are often lifelong. Doctors who easily diagnosed disability became popular. In 2008, only about one in five West Virginians received Supplemental Security (SSI) payments for disability, but a decade later, the state had the highest percentage of citizens on disability anywhere in America, almost 30 percent.[11]

Was it a coincidence that by the end of 2018, West Virginia also led America in deaths from drug overdoses with a rate two and a half times greater than overall in America?[12] Was it a coincidence that a few physicians wrote twenty-one million prescriptions for narcotics in a town in West Virginia with only thirty-two hundred citizens?[13] Was it a coincidence that between 2008 and 2018, two pharmacies a few hundred yards apart in the town of Williamson received more than twenty million pills for hydrocodone and oxycodone, more than six thousand five hundred pills per citizen?

In responding to a lawsuit against it, a national distributor of such pills claimed it hadn't noticed. But there is no plausible deniability here. For example, clerks in a Walgreen's store in Port Richey, Florida, could not believe how many oxycodone pills the store was getting: more than thirty-two hundred bottles a month for a town with far less than that many people.[14] Prosecutors later charged the store and chain with creating a "public nuisance" by failing to monitor its sales of such powerful drugs.

It is no surprise, then, that many West Virginians addicted to alcohol and drugs lived on the edge. Global capitalism had left them behind and Big Pharma and Big Alcohol stepped in to supply them with the means to self-medicate. Oxycontin became the soma of their brave new world.

Part of the problem of drug abuse in West Virginia was existential: people were bored and lacked the sense of purpose that a good career brings. A study forty years ago in public health sought to determine why middle-class teenagers in rural towns engaged in binge drinking and risky sex. The answer that emerged was that many such teenagers had little to do on weekends. Most weekends, they drove around in cars and trucks, parked and talked, and eventually, almost everyone started drinking and engaging in risky behavior. Boredom and the easy availability of alcohol and drugs led to unplanned pregnancies. In contrast, middle-class students in rich suburbs, engaged in time-consuming athletics such as competitive swimming or debate clubs, rarely had similar problems. Like teenagers who turn to beer and sex for stimulation, people trapped in rust-belt towns in West Virginia and along the Ohio River escaped into video games, the internet, alcohol, and drugs.

If proponents of globalism and open markets prevail, nothing will change for small, rural towns in America (or for rural Europe) for decades to come. That leaves Millennials in West Virginia with few options for long-term economic security, especially as more employers switch from defined-benefit pensions to defined-contribution pensions (if they offer pensions and health coverage at all).

JUSTICE, ADDICTION, AND OUR MOST VULNERABLE CITIZENS

Bioethics pays special attention to vulnerable populations, often used and abused in medical research, as shown by the Tuskegee Syphilis Study in Alabama. Run between 1929 and 1972 by the US Public Health Service, this study followed untreated syphilis in four hundred African American males, illiterate sharecroppers and descendants of slaves, who were the perfect subjects because their poverty, debt, and lack of education bound them to the land.

Social Justice advocates analyze how the basic structure of society (and changes in it) affect its most vulnerable citizens. They believe that whether you are overweight, experience daily temptation to drink alcohol, use crack cocaine, or inject heroin depends on which zip code you inhabit. They believe that structural inequalities involving access to good education, primary medical care, and intact families begin at birth and follow children into adulthood. Whether it's the pattern of prescriptions for opioids, the likelihood of being victimized by drunk drivers or gunshot wounds, or the opportunity to gamble with one's paycheck, a just society should protect its most vulnerable citizens from constant temptation and exploitation.

BIG REHAB

We've given the pharmaceutical industry the pejorative label "Big Pharma," and the alcohol industry deserves to be likewise labeled as "Big Alcohol." What, then, about "Big Rehab"? Social Justice theorists also differ in looking at how patterns of reimbursement may not cure the problem but make it worse. Why, they ask, do so many people enter rehab centers multiple times? Why do some centers discharge clients without any way to get legal prescriptions for their maintenance medications? Is it because they want clients to relapse, so they can get their fees again?

Recall the discussion from chapter 3 about money and reimbursement.

In Palm Beach County, Florida, substance abuse centers are a $1 billion industry, and in the same county, two people overdose on opioids every day.[15] At one center in Delray Beach, Florida, a center refused to give a client her legally prescribed drugs when she left, forcing her to score drugs illegally.[16]

South Florida in particular became the center of systematic, rampant fraud against companies issuing medical insurance policies in 2017. According to a local district attorney, rehab centers there widely encouraged a "lethal cycle of intentional failure."

UTAH VERSUS NEVADA

Can the structure of a state inhibit alcoholism while a nearby one encourages it? Consider Utah versus Nevada. Victor Fuchs in *Who Shall Live? Health, Economics, and Social Choice* compared morbidity and mortality in these states.[17] He documented that those living in Nevada had rates of alcoholism and cancer far higher than in Utah.

The Social Justice model argues that you can't simply analyze drinking or using narcotics just inside the user: sometimes you need to step back and ask why so many like him exist. Obviously, the hostility of the Church of Latter-day Saints to alcohol, drugs, and tobacco enabled Utahans to live longer, healthier lives than Nevadans, with the latter's casinos, prostitution, and tolerance of alcohol and narcotics.

Social Justice theorists analyze how public policy allows or inhibits addiction. For example, European countries kept a tight grip on prescriptions for opioids, so they did not have North America's problems. To the family of an addicted twenty-year-old son, it might seem like it's just his choice to keep using, but from ten thousand feet above, we can ask why he got a prescription for Oxycontin in the first place, why it was so easy for him to get more, and why it was later easy for him to get cheap fentanyl on the streets.

HOW THE MASS MEDIA PORTRAYS ALCOHOLISM AND ADDICTION

Social Justice theorists critique the images of heavy drinkers and addicted users in the mass media. Photojournalist Ryan Christopher Jones argues that our images of people dependent on alcohol and narcotics are dominated by those of poor people living in wretched conditions.[18] In fact, he argues, most addicted people live in ordinary homes, even rich homes, and not the squalid conditions under an underpass in which they are so often depicted.

The disease model of alcoholism/addiction—as an inexorable juggernaut careening down to rock bottom—dominates the mass media. Such tropes prevent everyone from trying, or accepting, other models for treating addiction and alcoholism.

Some Social Justice theorists emphasize how many of our standardized pictures of addicted people are racist. More and more, leading figures, such as Baltimore's district attorney Marilyn Mosby, are accepting the view that arresting millions of black people on felony charges for possession of marijuana dooms these millions to a life of unemployment, menial labor, harassment by parole officers, which lead to depression, anger, and despair, all, in turn, leading to escape into harder drugs.[19] Despite similar patterns of use, African Americans are four times more likely to be arrested for possession of marijuana than whites.[20]

Racism does seem to infect many stories about addiction. In many news reports, accounts of addictions by parents of white, middle-class adults in their twenties present the cases as breaking news. The underlying message is that we expect this in inner-city ghettoes, not in white suburbia. In fact, deaths from opioid overdoses in the last two decades have overwhelmingly been among white people. Although American media may focus on whites, addicted black people constitute only 12 percent of American deaths in this category— which is roughly equivalent to their percentage in the overall population.[21] Thus, overdose deaths in America are largely a problem among whites.

ADDICTION, CRIMINALIZATION, AND THE MOST VULNERABLE

As a percentage of its population, the United States jails more of its citizens than any other developed country on earth. In 2016, the United States had more than 1.5 million people in state or federal jail, the largest number of prisoners in the world.[22] With the 600,000-plus prisoners in state and federal jails, in 2016 more than 10 million Americans have spent time in local and county jails.

As mentioned, although America has only 4.4 percent of the world's popu- lation, it consumes most of its opiates.[23] It also imprisons a higher percentage of its population than any other country in the world. Is there any relationship between these two awful statistics? Probably.

Inside prisons, many of America's two million prisoners suffer from opioid addiction or OUD. How do we know this? One study discovered that released prisoners carry ten times the risk of overdose death than the general population.[24] One noted expert in addiction among prisoners concluded, "Over the past decade, the evolving opioid epidemic has most likely contributed to an increasing proportion of people in correctional facilities who have OUD."[25]

Almost no prisoners get programs to help them taper usage before entering. Almost none get medication-substitution therapy inside. Almost none get any counseling there about AUD or OUD. Is it any wonder that, upon release, so many immediately relapse? Are our policies about alcohol and opiates part of our problem of mass incarceration? Is our problem of mass incarceration part of our AUD/OUD epidemic? The answer is "yes" to both.

Sometimes the general public expresses mean attitudes toward prisoners, arguing that for their heinous crimes, they deserve to suffer inside locked doors. As such, they claim, giving prisoners nice food, expensive medical treatment, and other privileges is wasteful and wrong. And if alcoholics and opiate addicts committed crimes that landed them in prison, and if they then must go through hard detoxification, well, "They deserve what they get." Such harsh attitudes almost guarantee a cycle of continued abuse of alcohol and opiates.

One of the biggest goals of Social Justice theorists is to switch national policy from criminalization of AUD and OUD to treatment. Like Harm Reduction advocates, Social Justice model advocates believe that incarcerating millions of Americans for possessing marijuana or selling it has been a colossal mistake. With this thinking, Portugal in 2001 implemented (what Rawls would call) "a more just basic structure" when it decriminalized almost all drugs.

Moreover, America's long War on Drugs has jailed people of color at many times the rate of whites. And to what end? A felony conviction for drugs condemns any ex-prisoner to a lifetime of menial labor or unemployment because, in this day of instant background checks, no one can hide such convictions, and few employers will hire people with drug convictions.[26] For all these reasons, many in Europe regard America's burgeoning prisons, filled with people of color ruined by drug convictions, as moral stains for incarcerating so many people but also jailing so many people of color and so many for using drugs.

In 2018, a thirty-two-year-old man in Massachusetts successfully sued Essex

County in that state to provide him with methadone inside prison and argued that depriving him of it was cruel and unusual punishment as well as discrimination against a person with a disability (the disease of OUD).[27]

Stephanie DiPierro of Massachusetts became addicted to opiates as a teenager after her mother died of cancer around 1999. In 2005, she started a substitute-medication program, getting methadone each day at a clinic. She later committed fraud to get disability and earned a year in prison for doing so. Before entering prison, she sued the Federal Bureau of Prisons to obtain methadone for her year in prison, fearing that if she didn't get it, she would emerge out of control over her addiction and "relapse, overdose, and die."[28]

The Massachusetts prison system estimates that of its 180,000 inmates, 72,000 suffer from AUD or OUD. That system allows use of methadone to help incoming inmates detox but does not allow its use in prison as ongoing, medication-substitution treatment. DiPierro's lawsuit claimed that medication-assisted treatment for opiate addiction is now the standard of care and that denying her that treatment violated her rights both as an American and as a person with a disability.

It would be so much more humane, much less expensive, and much more just to aggressively teach these inmates to control their worst symptoms. As New York mayor Michael Bloomberg noted in an op-ed essay, "Helping prisoners overcome their addiction is crucial to helping them abstain upon release, yet few states offer medication-substitution therapy to prisoners. That treatment, when linked to addiction services after release, boosts the odds of putting their lives back together and reduces the likelihood that they will return to crime."[29] To his credit, Bloomberg preceded his op-ed with a $50 million donation to combat opioid-overdose deaths.[30]

Social Justice theorists argue that it's much cheaper to treat addicts than to jail them. Jailing victims of AUD/OUD and marijuana usage is exorbitant for taxpayers, costing ten times the amount of treatment in rehab, which (as we've seen) is not cheap. Portugal spends about $10 a citizen on drug prevention and treatment, whereas in contrast, by some estimates, America spends as much as $10,000 per household on implementing its drug policies (which includes imprisonment for possession of minor drugs such as marijuana).[31]

ALCOHOL, VULNERABLE POPULATIONS, AND SOCIAL STRUCTURE

As noted, and according to a study by the Centers for Disease Control released in 2018, thirty-seven million American adults binge drink at least once a week, consuming seven drinks per binge. In terms of alcohol sold, that is *seventeen billion* drinks a year.[32] Who benefits from this pattern of drinking? Obviously, the alcohol industry, which wants to keep sales continuing and growing.

When one looks at how America's structure supports alcoholism and addiction, some numbers are impressive: seventeen billion drinks consumed in binge drinking; $35 billion spent treating alcoholism and addiction; twenty-three million Americans suffering from some kind of opiate dependence; and $7.4 billion spent in 2012 on prescriptions for opiates (up from $2.3 billion in 1999).[33] Although the overall number of prescriptions for opiates has declined since 2012, profits have still been vast for prescriptions for benzodiazepines, morphine, fentanyl, codeine, and related narcotics. Seventeen years before, Americans spent $121 billion on prescription drugs, but by 2018, this figure had tripled to $360 billion.[34] Again, Big Pharma and Big Alcohol benefit from such consumption.

How the structure of society makes alcohol available, and how it makes it seem desirable to drink, matters greatly as to how many people in that society become heavy drinkers. For example, according to the World Health Organization in 2018, during the previous twelve months almost 90 percent of Irish males consumed alcohol, whereas in Egypt, Iran, and Jordan, due to disdain for alcohol in Islam, the corresponding figure was 4–6 percent.[35]

Consider a bad social structure in North America's past: In the first half of the nineteenth century, Americans drank astonishing amounts of gin and whiskey, which are far more dangerous than wine and beer, averaging *six to seven gallons* of alcohol every year.[36] The resulting drunkenness, especially of men, led to an epidemic of domestic violence, early death, and unemployment. Alcoholism among so many males led feminists such as Carrie Nation to agitate for the ban on alcohol that came with the US Constitution's Eighteenth Amendment.

Today, in almost every city and town in America and on every weekend night, police know where bars are concentrated. It may be a mile-long strip of a highway, where restaurants serve alcohol at either bars or tables. It may be down some remote road at the county line.

Wherever these establishments are, most patrons drive to them, and so at closing, most must drive home. If a normal male after two drinks in an hour has a blood alcohol level of .08 for drivers over twenty-one, then almost everyone leaving these bars is unable to legally drive and is dangerous. If a person is one of the one in seven patrons who binge drinks every week, then that person is a lethal driver.

Why don't police subject every driver leaving these places to sobriety tests?

If they did, everyone would deserve arrest for DWI. These establishments would then lose money. Then their owners would complain to local politicians and withhold future contributions to the campaigns of those politicians. Citizens would also be enraged at the new intolerance of their long-standing habit of drunk driving. Any police officer who took the initiative and checked everyone driving from a bar at closing would likely be reassigned to other duties.

Notice that two facts are not in dispute: first, most people driving from bars at closing are legally drunk; second, when they drive drunk, they're dangerous.

Why do we tolerate the resulting carnage from drunk drivers? If we use the concept of the exposure effect, we know that releasing a million drunk drivers every Friday and Saturday night will result in a predictable number of car crashes, injuries and deaths. Yet we do tolerate this alcohol-fueled carnage. Why? For Social Justice theorists, it's because Big Alcohol and the restaurants and bars it serves make so much money from our present system.

Alcohol can also impose a different kind of injustice simply in the fact that its pervasive use puts those with a low physical tolerance of it at a disadvantage. Drinking is deeply woven into American life. At holiday parties and business meals, heavy consumption of alcohol is the norm. Ditto for most college campuses on weekend nights. But because some individuals are relatively insensitive to alcohol, whereas others are highly sensitive, the consumption of alcohol can benefit some while hurting others. In any arena, whether it is about sexual conquest or business advancement, if everyone is expected to match others in finishing drinks per round, some will be at a great disadvantage.

SOCIAL JUSTICE AND BIG PHARMA

What Rawls could not have foreseen was how the pharmaceutical industry became so powerful in protecting its interests. How powerful? How profitable? According to one source, the top ten pharmaceutical companies in America in 2002 made more profits together than the *combined profits of all the other 490 companies in the Fortune 500.*[37]

What are the chances that such an industry won't do everything in its power to maintain its profits? This certainly explains why Big Pharma has more lobbyists in Washington, DC, and state capitols, and better-paid lobbyists than those of the National Rifle Association, American Medical Association, and National Farm Bureau combined. This also explains why Big Pharma employs many well-paid "pharmacy representatives" who give medical students and physicians free trips and goodies in return for prescribing their brand-name drugs, a corruption well explained in Carl Elliott's *White Coat, Black Hat.*[38]

It is no surprise, then, that congressmen who help Big Pharma often leave Congress for lucrative jobs in the same industry. Former committee chairman Billy Tauzin, a Louisiana congressman, went to work for pharmaceutical companies after shepherding through a bill to expand Medicare's coverage for prescription drugs, the so-called "donut hole" bill.[39]

In the United States, Canada, and Great Britain, we have a system where people get drugs by prescription and pay very little for their drugs. The real costs are paid through premiums of group plans for insurance or through taxes. Treatment for alcoholism and addiction is funded the same way. All of this enormously benefits Big Pharma and those who mop up after its messes.

Given the power of Big Pharma in America—and, indeed, internationally—is there any likelihood that its influence will diminish soon? The same could also be asked for Big Alcohol.

SOCIAL JUSTICE FROM OTHER MODELS

Social Justice model advocates believe that all other models miss the big picture and therefore their solutions are piecemeal. For example, the Harm Reduction model is great, but don't we want to know why in some cultures so much more harm reduction is needed than in others? Why did so few Portuguese become addicted to opiates versus Americans? If a million more Americans were addicted than Portuguese, is Harm Reduction the real answer?

Libertarians hate the perspective of the Social Justice model. Rich libertarians spend lots of money funding scholars and institutes that emphasize the individual. An example is revealing. For Social Justice theorists, Denmark is the happiest country in the world. It has high taxes but also cradle-to-grave health care for all, including long-term care and dentistry, as well as free access to excellent education, including college. With a thirty-seven-hour work week, it also offers parents of a new baby fifty-two weeks paid parental leave (between the two of them) to care for the newborn. Such a stress-free work-life balance makes Danes consistently rank as the happiest on the planet. The structure of Danish society minimizes the gap in life prospects between rich and poor, creating happiness.

In contrast, libertarians argue that the lack of happiness, or presence of it, is all in our heads. They fund studies that reflect this viewpoint. No matter how poor your life prospects, they say, you can always look on the bright side.

Even in the most unjust societies, if people adopt the right attitude, they can be happy.[40]

Of course, Social Justice theorists retort, this is a strategy for keeping people docile. It is a strategy for keeping them from coming together in unions or large voting masses. It is a strategy that serves to perpetuate economic inequality. It also seems ludicrous in places such as North Korea or in devastated countries of South America and the Middle East.

The Harm Reduction model also sees addiction very differently from Social Justice. If you have a patient who is struggling with alcoholism or addiction, about to kill himself because he hates himself and his family hates his behavior, the Social Justice model doesn't offer you any immediate help. If you are going through withdrawal, Social Justice doesn't say much about your need for medication substitution. For Harm Reductionists, the Social Justice model does very little in actually reducing harm for the individual.

For Harm Reduction, saying we can't solve addiction until we create a just society where citizens don't feel the need for drugs or alcohol is like saying we can't work to rid ourselves of the vestiges of racial segregation until we have a perfect society. Such either-or thinking flies in the face of Harm Reduction's incrementalism.

If you are trying to place responsibility for why someone misbehaves with alcohol or drugs, the Social Justice model seems to place the blame on society's structure, not on personal choices. In that way, Kantians and AA/NA think it misguided at best and useless at worst.

The Social Justice model is the ultimate expression of the "It takes a village to raise a child" philosophy made famous by Hillary Clinton. And the ancient Greeks were correct that it is much easier to be a good person in a good society that raises good children, praises their achievements, has good role models, and provides satisfying lives for them.

Can you be a good person in a bad society? Yes, it's possible, but as Socrates, Plato, and Aristotle argued, it's far easier to be a good person in a just society. Can a college student live alcohol and drug free in the modern world? Yes, it's possible, but much in the structure of her society is pulling her downstream. Ideally, colleges should immunize students against the dangers of alcohol and drugs, rather than letting them swim in the wrong streams until they find themselves over their heads. For a century, colleges have turned a blind eye to underage and excessive drinking in fraternities on campus. Only when students *died* did some begin to take action.

Nevertheless, one can imagine social worker Jack Trimpey's response: "Oh, yeah, I've got a patient with a gun to his head because he hates being an addict and what it's done to his family, and you're telling me the only real solution for him is to completely overhaul the structure of society?"[41]

CONCLUSIONS

It is silly to analyze the causes and prevention of alcoholism and addiction without a wider sociological view about the structure of a society. Although it is much harder to change the basic structure of a society, it is not impossible. If nothing else, paying attention to the injustices of some societies and how they exploit the vulnerable should make us more compassionate about those who fail and become addicted.

Augustine saw human life as trying to swim upstream in a powerful river of sin; hence, we are doomed to drown unless we get help from God or a supportive church. Are Americans not also doomed to fail in a similar river of alcohol and narcotics? They are encouraged to consume alcohol after work and to take opiates after sports injuries, after dental surgery, and after back injuries. As for prevention and education, do students get anything more than passing sermons to help them navigate these treacherous waters?

But let's face it: The Social Justice model is not a practical one for addiction counselors. Rather, it's more of a different lens through which to view our epidemic of addiction to opiates and alcohol. Privately, Social Justice advocates admit that society is unlikely to change for the better very soon.

Right now, workers' consciousness of the causes of their plight is low, easily manipulated by conservative mass media. The financially elite 1 percent continue to prosper: according to Robert Reich, 95 percent of the financial gains since 2009 went to the top 1 percent by net worth. For example, "The fortunes of a dozen 2009 Davos attendees have soared by a combined $175 billion, even as median U.S. household wealth has stagnated, a Bloomberg analysis found."[42]

Along the way, something has gone profoundly wrong in communities such as Vancouver or Kensington or indeed with all the heroin addicts living under bridges in Tehran. And regardless of what caused them to fall into such a life, a just society should help them.

Let's also face another truth: Where and how you live matters a lot in whether you become addicted or live a long life. A 2019 study by researchers at NYU School of Medicine analyzed health data by zip codes in the five hundred largest US cities and found that life expectancy varied by as much as thirty years between neighborhoods in the same city.[43] On average, those in the best zip codes lived twenty years more than those in the worst. When you think about it, these are astonishing statistics; they imply that if you could somehow move someone in Philadelphia from Kensington to Chestnut Hill, and if they lived the rest of their life in Chestnut Hill, they would likely live twenty more years.[44]

Summary of the Social Justice Model

Underlying cause: The distribution of wealth, income, and meaningful employment in a society affects its rates of alcoholism and addiction. Those with power use alcohol and drugs to manipulate poor people, both in selling them these evils and in ignoring the consequences of their substance abuse. The institutions of society can be structured to minimize exposure to addiction and alcohol, as Utah shows, and can minimize the harm of usage, as Portugal shows. Opiates were hard to get in Portugal but too accessible in America. Whether a society criminalizes low-level drugs, such as marijuana, alcohol, and nicotine, affects how people use and what happens to users. Access to treatment affects whether and how quickly users recover and whether they can function in society while addicted and working.

Treatment: Because large-scale alcoholism and addiction are symptoms of an unjust society, it is the obligation of a just society to provide facilities that prevent overdoses and reduce harm. Likewise, society should provide a range of treatments to help people recover. Society should create a just environment where citizens from birth have equal opportunities to be happy and to live meaningful lives.

Other models: Seeing addiction just as a problem of small units—whether inside the individual's body and mind or outside with his behavior or within the context of his family and peers—only goes so far in explaining why addiction runs so rampant in some societies but is mostly absent in others. A larger, corrective view is needed to balance individualistic models.

Responsibility: Although addicted people may initially have some free will and responsibility for substance abuse, they are less free than they think. The cards are stacked against them: Temptation is everywhere, and when people succumb, the dominate ideology of blaming the victim occurs. An unjust society is ultimately responsible for causing, tolerating, and not correcting mass addiction and alcoholism. Society can be structured to provide universal, free access to treatment, especially for people under twenty and in prison.

Family matters: Caught in the maw of an unjust society that encourages and tolerates mass addiction, families can try to practice harm reduction and tolerance and help where they can. Ultimately, the powerful forces aligned against them—from powerful new drugs to staggering profits for pharmaceutical companies—may be too much for addicted people to resist and families should not blame themselves for these problems.

THE SEVEN
APPROACHES AND
SUPER-POT

I n this chapter, I utilize ideas from most of the seven approaches discussed
previously to question the wisdom of the sudden, widespread legalization
of marijuana. After this chapter, the book concludes with ten insights from the
best of the seven models.

After five years of legalization in Colorado, statistics show that 90 percent of
its citizens can handle marijuana. That is especially true for well-off baby
boomers who, as tourists, sample a little pot while vacationing there, as well as
for Denverites who smoke on weekends at their cabins in the Rockies.
Although visits to emergency rooms have increased for those who react poorly
to pot, no one has died from cannabis (some may have died or killed others
while driving stoned, but that can't be proved, in part because traces of pot
stay in blood for thirty days).

But what about the 5–10 percent of people in Colorado, Washington State,
California, the District of Columbia, and Canada who may be vulnerable to
dependency or worse? Are we going to repeat our experiment with mass prescribing of opiates, only to later understand the dire consequences on poor,
immature adolescents? It would appear so.

THE EXPOSURE EFFECT

Over 28 million Americans and 38 million Canadians are now in an experiment where all forms of marijuana have suddenly been legalized, an experiment of great interest to Social Justice analysts. In public health, the "exposure

effect" is what happens when a previously naive population is abruptly exposed to a new substance, like the first exposure of rum to Native Alaskans. What will happen with this experiment?

Take a formerly dry county, such as Winston County in north Alabama, and follow what happened when alcohol suddenly became legal to buy: a small percentage, perhaps 1 percent of its citizens, who had never been exposed to alcohol, suddenly became alcoholics.

For advocates of the Social Justice or Harm Reduction models, why they do so is not important. What we know is that if you expose a population to a new, addictive substance—whether it's Iranians exposed to cheap heroin, young Mexican women exposed to fentanyl, or teetotalers exposed to booze—some previously nonaddicted, vulnerable citizens become addicted. Although we cannot predict which at-risk individuals will succumb, we can predict the numbers.

The exposure effect allows us to quantify structural changes in the delivery of addictive substances. If Purdue Pharma hires six hundred drug reps to push Oxycontin in big dosages to a million American physicians who are treating twenty million patients, we can predict that, say, at least two hundred thousand Americans will become addicted. The exact formula or numbers aren't important here; what is important is the concept: introducing a new, potentially addictive substance has a downside, especially for a small percentage of vulnerable people.

BEER THEN AND NOW

As a freshman in college, I could only drink near beer (a watered-down concoction that was at most 2 percent alcohol by volume) and only at a few bars or restaurants in town. Many students, following these same restrictions, managed to get drunk on it, although, due to the great volume needed to reach that state, they often got sick by that time.

In retrospect, having only near beer available to students was a Harm Reduction model tactic, and it seems that even eighteen-year-olds could drink it. Freshmen were also not allowed to have cars on campus, so no one drove home drunk. From a Social Justice model perspective, this was benign paternalism.

Biochemists say adult livers can safely process one regular beer in an hour. What is a regular beer? It is a traditional beer, which contains 4–6 percent alcohol by volume. Budweiser, for example, is 5 percent.

Not all beers are the same, especially the increasingly popular craft beers made by local breweries. With new craft beers, not all beers are equal. For example, Duvel Belgian Ale (red) is 8 percent alcohol and Samuel Adams Triple Bock is 15 percent.[1] Some home beer brewers claim to have achieved an even higher percent. So what has been quietly occurring is that the beer-wine-liquor industry has been creating more and more potent products.

Something else happened at my college during this time. Fraternities would throw parties and invite girls from sororities, especially after freshmen rush. They would buy a new trashcan and fill it with Hawaiian punch. A senior would drive to the ABC store and buy a gallon of tasteless grain alcohol, which can be as much as 95 percent alcohol, to be added to the punch. One small cup of the resulting powerful, tangy-tasting drink could easily inebriate a fresh-men girl, and two to three cups could make her pass out, which some did at their peril.

Today, in retail stores selling recreational marijuana in Colorado and Washington, the amount of delta-9-tetrahydrocannabinol (THC), the active ingredient in the products sold, ranges from 12 percent to 29 percent. THC can further be extracted from leaves and concentrated into a wax or oil, which can then be smoked. The result can have a THC content as high as 90 percent. Some marijuana clubs in Barcelona, Spain, where anyone can smoke on the premises, sell such products.[2]

Amazingly, cannabis has rapidly become more potent not over decades but over a few years. When I was in college in the late 1960s, the typical marijuana plant had a THC content of 5 percent.[3]

Will frat parties in states with legal pot soon have pot candy with 30 percent THC? Similar vaping sticks? Are eighteen-year-old freshmen guys and girls mature enough to make good decisions after ingesting such stuff? Will patterns repeat, where twenty-one-year-olds buy for all the kids under twenty-one, as has happened for a century in fraternities? What if someone buys hashish oil with 90 percent THC?

FRAMING EFFECTS

Before answering that question, consider a problem with the way many people frame the new, massive legalization of cannabis. Remember that the first step in a debate is often how the issue is framed, and accepting the wrong frame can bias the entire discussion.

The problem is that people think that the new marijuana is like the old marijuana of the 1960s, but, of course, it's not. "People like to romanticize the hippie generation and the pot-smoking that went on then," says one expert.[4] They think the new marijuana is like what they previously smoked in their college days—that is, the equivalent of near beer.

But smoking highly potent pot on campuses today is like going to a fraternity party where the main intoxicant is pot with 30 percent THC. Are kids really prepared to smoke or vape pot with that amount of THC? What about 90 percent THC? How do we prevent underage teenagers from getting it? At what age is the brain adult enough to handle daily smoking of such potent stuff? Not eighteen.

CANNABIS AND YOUNG BRAINS[5]

The American Academy of Pediatrics worries about the effects of widespread legalization of marijuana on adolescents. Its conclusions partly come from the Neuroscience model. In January 2015, it warned, "For adolescents, marijuana can impair memory and concentration, interfering with learning, and is linked to lower odds of completing high school or obtaining a college degree. . . . Regular use is . . . linked to psychological problems, poorer lung health, and a higher likelihood of drug dependence in adulthood."[6]

As we've seen, the adolescent brain is still developing and susceptible to foolish risk-taking and addiction. An important study in New Zealand found strong evidence that weekly consumption of even low-grade marijuana as teenagers damages developing brains.

In this study, researchers tested the IQ of more than one thousand thirteen-year-olds who had never before used. The researchers retested the IQs of the same people when they were thirty-eight. Those who used marijuana heavily during their teens—who met the criteria for cannabis dependence—and who continued as adults, by age thirty-eight had lost an average of eight points of IQ compared to those who had never used marijuana (who showed no decline in IQ).

And that study was where teenagers and adults smoked the *low*-THC pot of 1992–2017! How much damage will occur when teenagers smoke pot with THC levels of 90 percent?

Kenneth Davis and Mary Jeanne Kreek, two influential medical leaders in New York City, wrote an op-ed in the *New York Times* in 2019 as legislators fine-tuned a bill to legalize marijuana in New York. They cautioned Albany legislators to set age twenty-five as the minimal age for legally buying cannabis and urged them to restrict the THC content of legal cannabis to low levels and then to monitor what was sold.[7]

The Academy of Pediatrics also notes that MRIs of young recreational users of cannabis showed structural abnormalities in the brain associated with drug craving and dependence, as well as areas of reduced gray matter density in the prefrontal cortex. They noted that THC suppresses neurons in the information-processing part of the hippocampus and interferes with exchange of information among neurons, thus causing deterioration of learned behaviors.

The Academy likewise believes that a small percentage of adolescent daily marijuana users will become dependent on not only cannabis but also other drugs: "Research has shown that the younger an adolescent begins using drugs, including marijuana, the more likely it is that drug dependence or addiction will develop in adulthood."[8]

Predictably, some pediatricians are starting to see vaping as a gateway not just to cigarette smoking but also to use of other drugs.[9]

CANNABIS AS BIG BUSINESS

Consider vaping and e-cigarettes. Originally marketed as a harm-reductive alternative to cigarettes, everyone initially liked the idea. But Big Tobacco and Juul used deceptive marketing to target young people, making vaping taste like candy and seem safe. In 2019, states such as North Carolina sued Juul over its deceptive marketing and how it had misled adolescents.[10] Social Justice theorists are aghast at how Juul funded summer camps for kids and had its reps tell kids that vaping was safe.

Altria, which manufacturers Marlboro cigarettes and other brands, invested nearly $13 billion in Juul. Why? Some vapers transition to smoking cigarettes, and many cigarette smokers try vaping. Use of vaping among American teenagers spiked 78 percent from 2017 to 2018.[11] The harm of our foolish experiment with vaping became obvious in 2019, when the CDC said that more than twenty people had died from lung injuries associated with vaping and another 1,300 had serious lung injuries.[12]

The Brightfield Group, a team of scientists specializing in accurate data about market trends, forecasts that by 2022, sales of hemp-based products will be a *$22 billion industry in North America*.[13] Although as a party, Republicans opposed legalization of marijuana and voted to criminalize it, now that big money is coming from it, they're all for legalization.

For example, former Republican house majority leader John Boehner opposed legalizing marijuana while in office. When he left Congress in 2018, he got a lucrative job helping investors tap into industries selling marijuana. In 2018, he joined Acreage Holdings, a company lobbying for the medical use of pot and for changing the federal status of cannabis. In 2019, Boehner also became chair of the National Cannabis Roundtable, which lobbies for federal decriminalization of all marijuana products.

One predictor of how big and how fast the market will grow for legal marijuana is what happened overnight with marketing CBD oil, or cannabidiol, from the non-THC part of the hemp plant. One study predicts sales of this oil to be $22 billion by 2022.[14]

Marijuana Business Daily, a periodical devoted to the new gold rush and career counseling, advertises thousands of new jobs devoted to marketing, distributing, and selling marijuana. In North America, capital is now flooding into companies such as Weedmaps, an app showing customers the nearest store to buy cannabis products.

Many people have read the cutting-edge works of Canadian Malcolm Gladwell, a staff writer for the *New Yorker* and author of six books, such as *Outliers* and *The Tipping Point*, both on the *New York Times* best-seller lists. He is best known for revealing unexpected results of seemingly benign changes around us, usually by combining empirical investigations with academic research in the social sciences. Given all the above, Gladwell writes, "when powerful drugs are consumed by lots of people in new and untested ways, we have an obligation to try to figure out what will happen."[15]

LEGAL MARIJUANA AND THE MOST VULNERABLE

North America's sudden legalization of marijuana may be the biggest experiment in a century for vulnerable, mentally ill people, who may self-medicate themselves with marijuana the way people with schizophrenia self-medicate with nicotine (nicotine tends to inhibit hallucinations, for reasons unknown). But will this be a good or bad outcome for these people? Probably not good.

Given all the addicted people in Vancouver, was this the best time for Canada to legalize marijuana? At the time of my visit, they were six months into their experiment legalizing cannabis. Perhaps the best that can be said is that legal recreational marijuana, because of taxes, has been too expensive for most people addicted to opiates to buy.

We know that at least 1–2 percent of young people trying legal, recreational marijuana may become lifelong, heavy users with impaired motivation. Daily users are a whole different problem. A review of many studies in *Pharmacotherapy* in 2013 found that "cannabis is the most commonly used and abused illicit substance in the world. In the United States each year, approximately 6500 individuals begin to use marijuana daily, of whom 10–20% will develop cannabis dependence."[16] We should now start to replicate the New Zealand study and follow teenage daily users, testing their IQs now and ten, twenty, and thirty years from now. Only this time, they will have been smoking much more potent pot, so we can predict more damage to their IQs.

Overall, we don't now know what damage will occur to vulnerable people from mass legalization of super-pot. But now that it's available, we will, alas, discover it retrospectively.

CANNABIS AS DRUG-SUBSTITUTION THERAPY

New York, New Jersey, Pennsylvania, and Illinois by 2019 allowed high-dosage marijuana to be used to wean people from opioid addiction.[17] Is this a good idea?

In this book, I have been critical of the many unproven claims of Alcoholics and Narcotics Anonymous, but on one point, they may be correct. Several times in history, Harm Reductionists and others thought it safe to use a new drug to substitute for addiction to an old drug. Sigmund Freud relentlessly championed cocaine as a way of helping people recover from heroin addiction. Decades later, when physicians realized that cocaine was equally addictive, other physicians used morphine to wean physicians such as Freud and Halsted from cocaine.

New Hampshire has struggled with legalizing marijuana because it has a high rate of opioid addiction, causing 424 overdose deaths in 2017 and creating many orphans. Even some former addicts there oppose legalization of marijuana.[18] Although coastal states in America favor legalization, states of the Midwest—where alcohol and opiates have taken a heavy toll on the poor—are divided about its wisdom.

As a follower of Jack Trimpey might say, "Let's just focus on the drugs! And let's be careful not to fall down that rabbit hole of switching users from one addictive drug to another." Maybe the ultimate Coping model strategy should be to cope with life without any addictive drugs.

Now we have people arguing that marijuana can be used to wean people from addiction to alcohol or opiates. But let's be cautious here because, as emphasized, the new potent marijuana is not your grandfather's light stuff. It may prove to be as addictive as alcohol or opiates. And given the exposure effect of introducing high-potency cannabis to millions of new users, especially young users in high school and college, we know that a small percentage of new users will become dependent.

Narcotics Anonymous worries that substituting one drug for another doesn't solve the underlying problems of the person who is abusing opioids. It recognizes that most people can handle legal marijuana, but it worries about using high-potency marijuana for people with problems handling alcohol or opiates, as well as the exposure effect of widespread availability of high-potency marijuana to people at risk for addiction because of genes or social misfortune.[19] Narcotics Anonymous may be correct that the only true cure is no drugs, and even if lifelong abstinence is too lofty a goal, life without the daily use of an addictive drug should be the ultimate goal.

IS IT POLITICALLY INCORRECT TO SAY THE NEW POT IS DANGEROUS?

In the early 1980s, when HIV began slaying gay men and intravenous drug users, it was unclear how the virus spread. Some gay men claimed it did not spread through blood donations or sex and criticized those in public health who wanted to screen blood donated by gay men or close bath houses where unprotected sex occurred.

Because liberal-minded people appreciated that gay rights were new and hard won, they did not want to be seen as prudes, so they hesitated to back blood screening or closing bath houses. So fearful was the *New York Review of Books* that it was years before it admitted that HIV caused AIDS, that AIDS was often fatal, and that HIV spread through intravenous drug-sharing and sex.[20]

Today, no one wants to keep the draconian criminalization of marijuana, and no one denies that many middle-class citizens can handle a little recreational pot, especially on holidays. But such liberal tolerance opens the door to an "anything goes" approach to recreational pot and the vast monies it might create. The combination of these two forces—reluctance to seem prudish and desire for profits by big business—makes it difficult to argue that sudden, massive exposure to high-intensity pot is going to hurt vulnerable people.

And who is the most vulnerable of all, whether to opiates, alcohol, or cannabis? It's the human fetus inside a pregnant woman. We know there's no safe amount of alcohol for any pregnant woman to consume, but we know that millions of pregnant women still drink. Who knows how many kids exist with damaged IQs, motivational problems, or personality disorders stemming from their mother's drinking? Are we going to create similar problems with pot?

By the summer of 2019, one in fourteen pregnant women said they used pot within the last month, or 7 percent of all pregnant woman.[21] That's double the figure for 2002–2003. And because young women today obsess about their weight, they may be more likely to smoke a lot of pot than consume the calories of beer or wine.

Remember that most of the previous studies of damage to fetuses from pot were on the low-potency stuff. What is going on today with pot of 20 percent THC and pregnant women, we really don't know. And that should cause us to rethink what we've done.

Given all the above, it seems reasonable to conclude that customers should be at least age twenty-five to buy cannabis products and that the maximum legal THC content of products containing cannabis or its derivatives should be 25 percent.

TEN INSIGHTS FOR
FIGHTING OUR
EPIDEMICS

1. An ounce of prevention is worth a ton of treatment. From a Social Justice view, we need to create a society that discourages alcoholism and addiction in the first place. Powerful international corporations are pushing young people to drink alcohol and adopt lifestyles dependent on daily use of drugs. Starting in middle school with vaping, teachers and counselors need to teach students about the dangers facing them. How to do this is tricky, because past efforts were often too moralistic or focused on "Just Say No" strategies that seemed puritanical to many teenagers.

Dental students should learn to rarely give prescriptions for hydrocodone or opiates. Most people can get by with non-opiate painkillers. Both dental and medical schools need to fill the void in their typical curricula created by the lack of teaching about alcoholism and addiction, and they should be taught how previous dentists and physicians helped create the present epidemic.

2. Decriminalize addiction and don't punish addicts. Harm Reduction is right. To reduce overdose deaths upon release, treat addiction and alcoholism in prison, where counselors have a truly captive audience. Without treatment, addicted people and drinkers will resume old habits upon release but may not be able to handle the new fentanyl (or, if they use the old dosage without their previous tolerance, they may overdose).

3. Substitute therapy is necessary to reduce craving for those trying to quit. This is the great insight of Neuroscience. After using for a long time, not using

creates its own misery. Not the lack of a high—just the lack of a maintenance dose. Either you go through the pain of withdrawal all at once or you need a drug to reduce the craving.

4. Alcoholics Anonymous and Narcotics Anonymous are also correct about some things: First, people have the power to change. Some need the fellowship of others trying to do the same and the backing of calling on God. Second, the best way to recover, if possible, is without any drug substitution. In our past, too many substitute drugs were erroneously seen as non-addicting, or else counselors didn't understand how addicted people could get around them. Don't underestimate the ability of users to potentiate drugs in substitute therapy by combining them with other drugs. If marijuana is the substitute for opiates, watch out for high-THC cannabis piggy-backing on alcohol and cocaine or meth.

When a substitute drug is offered, the dosage should be tapered with the goal of cessation. Physicians should learn how to help patients taper and be reimbursed for doing so.

5. The fact that many heavy drinkers and drug users aren't lifetime abusers should give hope to families: Hang in there, chances are good that repeated attempts at therapy will converge with a more mature person who will eventually learn to cope better with alcohol and drugs. Maturing out is real and can create a new person.

6. Kant gets some things right: People have free will. To deny them such free will is to undercut reasons for entering therapy and, thus, chances of recovery. Although it is hard, the best way to quit is cold turkey.

On that matter, the late, leading drug researcher Ronald Siegel helped film producer Julia Philips (*Taxi Driver*) kick her addiction to cocaine. He advised her to go cold turkey and to take up running. "You'll get higher than you ever did on drugs," he told her.[1]

Kant is also right that, like being born again in Christianity, only the addicted person or drinker can ultimately decide to recover. It must come from within, not without. Counselors, partners, and families can nudge and cajole, but, ultimately, the person must want to change.

7. Social Justice has a point about the exposure effect. It is real.

Late in the summer of 2019, the *Washington Post* and HD Media won a years-long suit in court to release federally mandated reports on distribution of opioids.[2] We then learned why the drug companies, and even the DEA and Justice Department, had fought so long to keep this data from going public.

Over seven years, America's drug companies flooded the country not with hundreds of thousands of oxycodone and hydrocodone pills, not with millions of such pills, not even with a mere billion. The true number? *Seventy-six billion pills!*

How does that break down? Estimating that the US population during 2006–2012 averaged about 306 million, that is thirty-six Oxycontin pills, every year, for each man, woman, and child in our country. Curry County, Oregon; Walker County, Alabama; and Mingo County, West Virginia, had more than 140 opioid pills dispensed each year legally from pharmacies for every person in these counties.

During the years of both the Obama and the Trump administrations, something went horribly wrong. The power of the drug companies, by far the richest and most powerful industry in America, overwhelmed the Drug Enforcement Administration (DEA), the Justice Department, and the country. Everyone assumed that someone was in charge and monitoring the distribution of these terrible drugs, but no one was.

Who was distributing these drugs? Not just isolated, rogue pharmacies but also big chains, such as CVS, Walmart, and AmerisourceBergen. Walgreens, McKesson, and Cardinal Health distributed half of the seventy-six billion opiates.

It wasn't just Purdue Pharma that was guilty here. As the *Washington Post* found, "Just six companies distributed 75 percent of the pills during this period: McKesson Corp., Walgreens, Cardinal Health, AmerisourceBergen, CVS, and Walmart, according to an analysis of the database by the *Washington Post*. Three companies manufactured 88 percent of the opioids: SpecGx, a subsidiary of Mallinckrodt; Actavis Pharma; and Par Pharmaceutical, a subsidiary of Endo Pharmaceuticals."[3] Indeed, according to this analysis, Purdue Pharma came in merely fourth, with 3 percent of the market. Moreover, according to an analysis by the Associated Press, when the overall number of pills bought began to dip, manufacturers increased the potency of the pills sold, so users could maintain the same high with fewer pills.[4]

From a Social Justice perspective, offering Harm Reduction treatment, treating cravings, teaching better coping skills, studying genetics, or expanding Narcotics Anonymous does not matter *while the country is being flooded with opioid pills*. As one Stanford psychiatrist wrote, "Expanding health insurance and access to evidence-based treatment will indeed save lives, but health professionals are swimming up a waterfall if this isn't matched by strong drug supply control."[5]

8. From our discussion of the Genetics model, we should avoid genetic fatalism. We should also not exaggerate any correlations between a genetic variation and addiction or alcoholism. Let's be mindful of giving test takers a sick identity. Let's be mindful of the power of bad labels, a power already wielded harmfully on Native Americans.

Another lesson from Genetics is that we probably do process alcohol, marijuana, and other intoxicating substances in different ways, depending on which genes and genetic variations we inherit (and what our mother ingested when we were in the womb).

Heads up to college students: Just because someone you know tolerates something well doesn't mean you will. It pays to find out which camp fate has thrown you in.

9. From the Neuroscience and Harm Reduction models, let's make twenty-five the minimum age to buy marijuana products and make 25 percent the highest legal THC amount. Call this the 25/25 rule. Doing so will prevent damage to developing brains and lessen the chances of vulnerable people becoming addicted to pot.

10. From the Coping model, let's help heavy drinkers and addicted people by focusing on their main problem—which, as Jack Trimpey says, is drinking and/or using hard drugs. These people don't need to solve *all* of their problems to resolve their drinking/drug issues. Indeed, if they solved their problems with drinking or using drugs, some of their other problems might get better.

Finally, I close with a letter to a young college student in the manner of Richard Selzer's *Letters to a Young Surgeon* or David Foster Wallace's famous graduation address, *This Is Water*:

> My Dear Student,
>
> As you navigate your life through your college years and afterward in your twenties, know that dealing with addictive substances will be one of your greatest challenges. All around you, immensely powerful corporations will be trying to make you become dependent on what they're selling.
>
> Your generation has already become dependent—maybe we could even say "addicted"—to using Google to find anything and to living on social media platforms such as Instagram and Snapchat and on smartphones, so you know

what I'm talking about. Google, Apple, and Facebook make money from your use and dependence: lots and lots of money. Don't think they are your friends.

Everything around you in your culture says alcohol can be safely consumed, and this is the new normal for marijuana, too. Resist these marketing messages. In the same way, vaping is packaged with tasty flavors and candy colors and marketed as safe. It is not: nicotine is an addictive substance and one of the hardest drugs to kick. (Believe me: I smoked in college and greatly regret it now.)

When you get your wisdom teeth removed or have dental surgery, you don't need the prescription. Ninety percent of the time, Advil will do (and if doesn't, *then* fill the prescription or call the dentist for one). Don't take the pills as a way to get high. As Augustine said, this is jumping into a strong current that is very hard to swim against.

People will tell you that you're no fun if you don't drink with them or, worse, match their drinking. Ditto for using marijuana. Resist this bullshit. People who pressure you to drink alcohol or smoke dope are not your real friends.

So much pressure surrounds you to waste your money betting on sports or in casinos, to live on sugary sodas and overly processed foods, to spend most of your time in college on extracurricular activities rather than acquiring real knowledge.

Resist all this. Resist! Think for yourself. Be your own person. It will be hard, but in the long run, it will be worth it.

If nothing else, think of how much money you will save in life if you never buy tobacco, alcohol, pot, or opiates. If a normal person took all that money and put it in a piggy bank between the ages of twenty and forty, he or she would have enough to buy a home.

Most of all, Big Pharma will try to sell you drugs to sleep, not be nervous, stay thin, have sex, poop, avoid depression, overcome anxiety, be smarter, bulk up, and enhance your moods. Resist all this! Resist medicating your life.

NOTES

PREFACE

1. Vivek Murthy, "Ending the Opioid Epidemic—A Call to Action," *New England Journal of Medicine*, 375, no. 25 (December 22, 2016): 2413–15.

2. Alcohol contents of various alcoholic drinks and beers can be found at http://getdrunknotfat.com/alcohol-content-of-beer/. Popular light beers (Bud, Miller, Michelob) average about 4 percent alcohol.

3. "Ireland Has the Worst Rates in the World for Drinking during Pregnancy," *The Journal.ie.*, January 17, 2017, https://www.thejournal.ie/alcohol-pregnancy -ireland-3190327-Jan2017/.

4. For example, Paul Thomas, Leslie Jamison, Ann Johnston, Annie Grace, Judy Griesel, Marc Lewis, Maia Szalawitz, and others.

5. National Institute on Drug Abuse, "Principles of Drug Addiction Treatment: A Research-Based Guide (Third Edition)," https://www.drugabuse.gov/publications/ principles-drug-addiction-treatment-research-based-guide-third-edition/principles -effective-treatment (accessed May 18, 2019).

CHAPTER 1

1. Holly Hedegard, Ariali M. Miniño, and Margaret Warner, "Drug Overdose Deaths in the United States, 1999–2017," National Center for Health Statistics, https://www.cdc.gov/nchs/products/databriefs/db329.htm (accessed January 23, 2019).

2. Hawre Jalal et al., "Changing Dynamics of the Drug Overdose Epidemic in the United States from 1979 through 2016," *Science*, September 21, 2018, http:// science.sciencemag.org/content/sci/361/6408/eaau1184.full.pdf (accessed January 21, 2019).

3. Abby Goodnough et al., "Data Shows Drop in Drug Overdose Deaths for the First Time since 1990," *New York Times*, July 18, 2019, A17.

4. Beth Macy, "Four Ordinary People vs. Big Pharma," *New York Times*, July 21, 2019, SR10.

5. Dean Reynolds, "Overdoses Now Leading Cause of Death of Americans under 50," CBS News, June 6, 2017, https://www.cbsnews.com/news/overdoses-are-leading-cause-of-death-americans-under-50/ (accessed January 21, 2019); "Opioid Deaths by Age Group," Henry Kaiser Foundation, https://www.kff.org/other/state-indicator/opioid-overdose-deaths-by-age-group/?dataView=0&currentTimeframe=0&sortModel=%7B%22colId%22:%22Location%22,%22sort%22:%22asc%22%7D (accessed January 25, 2019).

6. Claire Galaforo, "Moms of Opioid Dead: 'Where Is the Outrage for Us?' " reprinted in *Tuscaloosa News*, January 29, 2019, A4.

7. Danny Hakim et al., "As Opioid Epidemic Grew, Family Spied New Market: Sacklers Saw an Opportunity to Profit from Addiction Treatments, Suits Reveal," *New York Times*, April 2, 2019, A11.

8. Adeel Hassan, "Deaths from Drug Use and Suicide Set Record in 2017, Analysis Shows," *New York Times*, March 8, 2019, A20. It is often difficult to know whether an overdose death was intentional or unintentional, so including suicide here can be helpful.

9. Gina Kolata, "The Biggest Losers," *New York Times*, 2017.

10. Kevin Rose, "How I Ditched My Phone and Unbroke My Brain," *New York Times*, February 23, 2019, B1–4.

11. Mike Snider, "Strung Out on Super Mario?" *USA Today*, May 29, 2019, A1.

12. Stephanie Labonville, "Opiate, Opioid, Narcotic—What's the Difference?" Injured Workers Pharmacy (IWP), March 29, 2017, http://info.iwpharmacy.com/opiate-opioid-narcotic-whats-the-difference.

13. Carl Elliott, *Better Than Well, American Medicine Meets the American Dream* (New York: W. W. Norton, 2003).

14. S. Podolsky et al., "Preying on Prescribers (and Their Patients)—Pharmaceutical Marketing, Iatrogenic Epidemics, and the Sackler Legacy," *New England Journal of Medicine*, 380, no. 19 (May 9, 2019): 1785–87.

15. T. Llyapustina and G. Alexander, "The Prescription Opioid Addiction and Abuse Epidemic: How It Came About and What We Can Do about It," *Pharmaceutical Journal*, June 11, 2015, https://www.pharmaceutical-journal.com//opinion/comment/the-prescription-opioid-addiction-and-abuse-epidemic-how-it-happened-and-what-we-can-do-about-it/20068579.fullarticle?firstPass=false.

16. Brian Mann, "Opioid Maker Charged with Fraud in Marketing Drug as Less Prone to Abuse," NPR News, April 10, 2019, https://www.npr.org/2019/04/10/711669778/opioid-maker-charged-with-fraud-in-marketing-drug-as-less-prone-to-abuse.

17. Llyapustina and Alexander, "The Prescription Opioid Addiction and Abuse Epidemic."

18. Katie Zezima and Lenny Bernstein, "'Hammer on the Abusers': Mass. Attorney General Alleges Purdue Pharma Tried to Shift Blame for Opioid Addiction," *Washington Post*, January 15, 2019.

19. Anthony Izaguirre and Geoff Mulvihill, "Five States Announce Lawsuits over Prescription Opioids," *Tuscaloosa News*, May 17, 2019, A4.

20. Katie Thomas, "Opioid Maker Agrees to Pay $225 Million to Settle Fraud Case Related to Fentanyl," *New York Times*, June 6, 2019, A19.

21. Colin Moynihan, "Guggenheim Targeted by Protesters for Accepting Money from Family with Oxycontin Ties," *New York Times*, February 9, 2019.

22. Anand Giridharadas, "Museums Must Reject Tainted Money," *New York Times*, May 19, 2019, SR9.

23. Because of allergies to latex, Nitrile gloves have become an industry standard for first responders. Nitrile feels a lot like latex but is allergy safe.

24. Mark Bradford, "Online Overdose: Frontotemporal Dementia," *60 Minutes*, May 5, 2019, https://www.cbs.com/shows/60_minutes/.

25. "'Record' Fentanyl Drug Bust Made at US-Mexico Border," BBC News, January 31, 2019, https://www.bbc.com/news/world-us-canada-47066311 (accessed February 3, 2019).

26. Anita Snow, "'Mexican Oxy' Pills in Southwest Raise Fentanyl Death Toll," *Medical Xpress*, February 14, 2019, https://medicalxpress.com/news/2019-02 -fentanyl-deaths-mexican-oxy-pills.html.

27. "The Opioid Epidemic Is No Time for Risky Pharmaceutical Marketing," Editorial, *Washington Post*, January 27, 2019.

28. Stefan Kertesz, "Turning the Tide or Riptide: The Changing Opioid Epidemic," *Substance Abuse* 38, no. 1 (2017): 3–8.

29. "The Opioid Epidemic Is No Time."

30. "Docs Among 60 Charged in Opioid Crackdown," *Ottawa Citizen*, April 18, 2019.

31. "The Addiction Crisis," *New York Times*, Special Supplement, December 27, 2017.

32. De Quincy's book and his friendship with William Coleridge, who also used opium, led to a claim that the use of opium, rampant in this period, created some of the best Romantic literature, a claim disputed by other scholars.

33. Did Mercury technically die of AIDS? Pneumonia secondary to end-stage HIV infection? Both combined with chronic substance abuse? It can be argued any of these ways.

34. Centers for Disease Control, "During Binges, U.S. Adults Have 17 Billion Drinks a Year," press release, March 16, 2018, https://www.cdc.gov/media/releases/ 2018/p0316-binge-drinking.html (accessed February 4, 2019).

35. "Alcohol Use Disorder: A Comparison between DSM–IV and DSM–5," National Institute on Alcohol Abuse and Alcoholism, https://www.niaaa.nih.gov/publi cations/brochures-and-fact-sheets/alcohol-use-disorder-comparison-between-dsm-

36. "Fact Sheet: Alcohol Use and Your Health," Centers for Disease Control, https://www.cdc.gov/alcohol/fact-sheets/alcohol-use.htm (accessed February 4, 2019).

37. World Health Organization (WHO), *Global Status Report on Alcohol* (Geneva: World Health Organization, 2004), http://www.who.int/substance_abuse/publica tions/global_status_report_2004_overview.pdf.

38. B. Grant et al., "Prevalence of 12-Month Alcohol Use, High-Risk Drinking, and *DSM-IV* Alcohol Use Disorder in the United States, 2001–2002 to 2012–2013: Results from the National Epidemiologic Survey on Alcohol and Related Conditions," *JAMA Psychiatry* 74, no. 9 (September 2017): 911–23.

39. "Does Drinking 1 Bottle of Wine a Week Raise Cancer Risk as Much as 10 Cigarettes?" *Marketwatch*, March 28, 2019, https://www.marketwatch.com/story/does -drinking-1-bottle-of-wine-a-week-raise-cancer-risk-as-much-as-10-cigarettes-2019 -03-28.

40. Abby Godnough, "Heroin Is Vanishing as Fentanyl Swamps Streets," *New York Times*, May 19, 2019.

41. S. H. Podolsky, D. Herzberg, and J. A. Greene, "Preying on Prescribers (and Their Patients)—Pharmaceutical Marketing, Iatrogenic Epidemics, and the Sackler Legacy," *New England Journal of Medicine* 380, no. 19 (May 9, 2019): 1785–87.

CHAPTER 2

1. For more, see "Psychiatry Epidemiology" at https://en.wikipedia.org/wiki/ Psychiatric_epidemiology.

2. Dan Levin, "A Weary Child's Plea: Become My Mom Again," *New York Times*, June 1, 2019, A1–18.

CHAPTER 3

1. Herbert Fingarette, "The Perils of Powell," *Harvard Law Review* 83, no. 4 (February 1970), 809.

2. "NIH Names Dr. George Koob Director of the National Institute on Alcohol Abuse and Alcoholism," National Institute on Alcohol Abuse and Alcoholism, press release, October 31, 2013, https://www.niaaa.nih.gov/news-events/news-releases/dr -george-koob-named-niaaa-director (accessed February 20, 2019).

3. B. A. Y. Cher, N. E. Morden, and E. Meara, "Medicaid Expansion and Pre-scription Trends: Opioids, Addiction Therapies, and Other Drugs," *Medical Care* 57, no. 3 (2019): 208–12.

4. Richardo Alonso-Zaldivar and Carla K. Johnson, "The New War on Drugs," *Birmingham News*, February 3, 2019.

5. Kyle Spencer, "Opioids on the Quad," *New York Times*, November 5, 2017, 24.

6. Jake Flanagin, "The Surprising Failure of 12 Steps," *The Atlantic*, March 5, 2014, https://www.theatlantic.com/health/archive/2014/03/the-surprising-failures-of-12-steps/284616/ (accessed February 2, 2019).

7. "America's Addiction Crisis," *New York Times*, Special Supplement, December 28, 2017.

8. Michael Corkery and Jessica Silver-Greenberg, "The Giant, under Attack," *New York Times*, December 28, 2017, F3.

9. Corkery and Silver-Greenberg, "The Giant, under Attack," F6.

10. Michael Smith, Jonathan Levin and Mark Bergen, "Why It Took Google So Long to Regulate Shady Rehab Center Ads," *Bloomberg News*, September 26, 2017.

11. Corkery and Silver-Greenberg, "The Giant, under Attack."

12. Terry Spencer, "Florida 'Pill Mills' Were the 'Gas on the Fire' of Opioid Crisis," *Tuscaloosa News*, July 21, 2019, A3.

13. Smith et al., "Why It Took Google So Long."

14. David Segal, "City of Addict Entrepreneurs," *New York Times*, December 27, 2018, F8–F12.

15. David Segal, "In Pursuit of Liquid Gold," *New York Times*, December 28, 2017, F12.

16. Danny Hakim et al., "As Opioid Epidemic Grew, Family Spied New Market: Sacklers Saw an Opportunity to Profit from Addiction Treatments, Suits Reveal," *New York Times*, April 2, 2019, A1.

17. David Segal, "The Mysterious 'Man in Blue,'" *New York Times*, December 27, 2018, F14.

18. Families can get some help by reading reviews of centers that treat addiction online—for example, https://www.rehabs.com/listings/bradford-health-services-2929092450/.

19. Smith et al., "Why It Took Google So Long."

20. See the chart in Smith et al., "Why It Took Google So Long."

21. Segal, "The Mysterious 'Man in Blue,'" F14–F15.

22. "Google Resumes Accepting Ads for Addiction Treatment Centers," Recovery Centers of America, August 14, 2018, https://recoverycentersofamerica.com/rca-news/google-resumes-accepting-ads-from-addiction-treatment-centers/. If you go on some sites, such as Narconon, a chat box will open and some may say, "Desiree from Narconon: Hello my name is Desiree. Are you looking for help for yourself or someone you know?" https://www.narconon.org/blog/did-portugal-really-legalize-all-drugs.html (accessed May 18, 2019).

23. Julie Carr Smyth, and Geoff Mulvihill, "Towns, Counties, Are Paying the Price for Opioid Crisis," *Birmingham News*, March 29, 2019, A15.

24. Herbert Fingarette, *Mapping Responsibility: Essays in Mind, Law, Myth, and Culture* (Chicago: Open Court, 2004), 49.

CHAPTER 4

1. Alcoholics Anonymous, *Alcoholics Anonymous: The Story of How Many Men and Women Have Recovered from Alcoholism*, 4th edition (New York: Alcoholics Anonymous World Services, 2001).

2. The term first appeared (in 1849) in the Swedish edition of *Alcoholismus Chronicus, or Chronic Alcohol Illness: A Contribution to the Study of Dyscrasias Based on My Personal Experience and the Experience of Others*, which was soon translated to German (1852) and later into English.

3. James R. Milam, *The Emergent Comprehensive Concept of Alcoholism* (self-published 1970; New York: Bantam, 1981).

4. James R. Milam and Katherine Ketchum, *Under the Influence: A Guide to the Myths and Realities of Alcoholism* (New York: Simon & Schuster, 1981).

5. Frank McCourt, *Angela's Ashes: A Memoir* (New York, Touchstone, 1999).

6. Alcoholics Anonymous World Services, Inc. (2016).

7. Kyle Spencer, "Opioids on the Quad," *New York Times*, November 5, 2017, 24.

8. Alcoholics Anonymous, *Alcoholics Anonymous*.

9. AA does not care which deity you posit and doesn't care that much about denominations and organized religions, but it does insist on being a theist—that is, believing in a god who takes a personal interest in how your life is going.

10. Alcoholics Anonymous, *Alcoholics Anonymous*, 35.

11. Quoted in Jake Flanagin, "The Surprising Failure of 12 Steps," *The Atlantic*, March 5, 2014, https://www.theatlantic.com/health/archive/2014/03/the-surprising-failures-of-12-steps/284616/ (accessed February 2, 2019).

12. Flanagin, "The Surprising Failure of 12 Steps."

13. "Bloody Mary" is the fourteenth episode in the ninth season of South Park. See https://en.wikipedia.org/wiki/Bloody_Mary_(South_Park) (retrieved January 27, 2019).

14. Lance Dodes, *The Sober Truth: Debunking the Bad Science Behind 12-Step Programs and the Rehab Industry* (Boston: Beacon Press, 2014), 53.

15. Fingarette became, like Peter Singer, one of the most controversial philosophers of his day because he deeply delved into actual problems around him while simultaneously applying insights from philosophy, comparative religion, and psychoanalysis to such problems. University of Texas professor Robert Solomon wrote that Fingarette "has long been one of the most original and provocative philosophers in America."

16. Herbert Fingarette, "The Perils of Powell," *Harvard Law Review* 83 (1970): 793–812.

17. Fingarette, "The Perils of Powell."

18. *Traynor v. Turnage*, 485 U.S. 535 (1988).

19. Fingarette, "The Perils of Powell," 797.

20. Herbert Fingarette, "Why We Should Reject the Disease Concept of Alcoholism," in *Controversies in the Addiction Field*, ed. Ruth C. Engs (Dububuqe, IA: Kendall-Hunt, 1990).

21. William Madsen, a professor of anthropology at Fingarette's university, was so incensed by Fingarette's views that he published a famous attack on them, *Defending the Disease: From Facts to Fingarette*. The news program *60 Minutes* later regretfully took Madsen's viewpoint in criticizing Mark and Linda Sobell, two pioneering psychology professors in addiction research, and implied that their model had killed some patients. In the early 1970s in California, the Sobells argued in studies that severe alcoholics who were taught to control, but not eliminate their drinking completely, fared better for the first two years after treatment than alcoholics who were urged only to abstain entirely. Their "findings were challenged . . . by Dr. Pendery and Dr. Maltzman, who charged that many of the controlled drinkers actually suffered serious relapses. Subsequently, some of the patients in the study filed a lawsuit seeking $96 million in damages stemming from the 'controlled drinking' treatment" (see Philip M. Boffey, "Panel Finds No Fraud by Alcohol Researchers," *New York Times*, September 11, 1984). The assumption behind the suit, of course, was that any result other than abstinence for life constituted failure of the experiment. What is important about the attacks on the Sobells and Fingarette is that champions of AA and neuroscience falsely painted them as Darth Vaders. The attackers knew about spontaneous remissions but refused to acknowledge them. The attack was so fierce as to make other researchers shy away from agreeing with or publicizing any view contrary to the received wisdom. Stanton Peele, one of the oldest and most famous psychologists specializing in treating alcoholism and addiction, investigated Fingarette's work and Madsen's attacks and concluded that Fingarette was correct about almost everything and that Madsen's attack was unprofessional, vicious, and personal. So here we are with treatment of alcoholism and addiction today, a $35 billion industry of urine testing and rehab centers, with even more billions spent on research into the brain. With that much money at stake, who is going to believe, much less publicize, facts that most drinkers and users can quit without being in any program? In some ways, the attacks on the Sobells and Fingarette resemble the attacks on Ignaz Semmelweis and his groundbreaking idea that childbed fever could be prevented by physicians washing their hands, with its corollary that by going from bed to bed in delivering babies, physicians were actually spreading the fever. The medical establishment could not accept this idea, and Semmelweis was condemned by his peers for his ideas, suffered severe anxiety attacks and depression, and died in an institution at age forty-seven.

22. Kavita Babu et al., "Prevention of Opioid Overdose," *New England Journal of Medicine* 380, no. 13 (June 6, 2019): 2251.

23. Caroline Knapp, *Drinking: A Love Affair* (New York: Dial Press, 1986), 22. In fact, Knapp's drinking led to her early death at age forty-two.

24. Amy Dresner, *My Fair Junkie: A Memoir of Getting Dirty and Staying Clean* (New York: Hatchette, 2017), 70–71.

25. Herbert Fingarette, "Self-Deception Needs No Explaining," *Philosophical Quarterly*, 48, no. 192 (1998): 289–300.

26. Maia Szalavitz, *Unbroken Brain: A Revolutionary Way of Understanding Addiction* (New York: Picador/St. Martin's Press, 2016), 189.

27. Some might go further and claim that a medical model requires an all-or-nothing diagnosis ("You either have cancer or you don't") and a description of necessary and sufficient conditions for the disease, such that each and every person fitting those conditions has the disease. But these additional requirements violate standard diagnoses of diseases treated by physicians, such as diabetes, which runs a spectrum of severity, or slow-growing prostate "cancer" in older men, which may or may not be the same cancer as the lethal, fast-growing kinds that can quickly spread to stage IV.

28. Sheldon Zimberg, *The Clinical Management of Alcoholism* (New York: Routledge, 1982).

29. Charles Winick, "Maturing Out of Addiction," United Nations Office on Drugs and Crime, January 1, 1962, https://www.unodc.org/unodc/en/data-and-analysis/bulletin/bulletin_1962-01-01_1_page002.html (accessed March 9, 2019).

30. G. D. Walters, "Spontaneous Remission from Alcohol, Tobacco, and Other Drug Use: Seeking Quantitative Answers to Qualitative Questions," *American Journal of Drug and Alcohol Abuse* 26, no. 3 (August 2000): 443–60.

31. Rumo Kato Price et al., "Remission from Drug Abuse over a 25-Year Period: Patterns of Remission and Treatment Use," *American Journal of Public Health* 91, no. 7 (July 2001): 1107–12.

32. R. B. Cutler and D. A. Fishbain, "Are Alcoholism Treatments Effective? The Project MATCH Data," *BMC Public Health* 14, no. 5 (2005): 75.

33. Deborah Dawson et al., "Recovery from DSM-IV Alcohol Dependence," *Addiction* 100, no. 3 (2005): 281–92.

CHAPTER 5

1. Nora Volkow et al., "Neurobiologic Advances from the Brain Model of Addiction," *New England Journal of Medicine* 374 (2016): 363–71.

2. I am indebted to Vanessa Bentley, a visiting professor at University of Alabama at Birmingham, 2018–2020, for pointing out Leshner's original article to me.

3. Alan Leshner, "Addiction Is a Brain Disease, and It Matters," *Science* 278, no. 5335 (October 3, 1997): 45–47.

4. "Alan I. Leshner," Wikipedia, https://en.wikipedia.org/wiki/Alan_I._Leshner.

5. Vivek Murthy, "Ending the Opioid Epidemic: A Call to Action," *New England Journal of Medicine* 375, no. 25 (December 22, 2016): 2413–15.

6. Neil Levy, "Addiction Is Not a Brain Disease (And It Matters)," *Frontiers in Psychiatry* 4, no. 24 (April 11, 2013).

7. Volkow et al., "Neurobiologic Advances," 364.

8. Carlton Erickson, *The Science of Addiction: From Neurobiology to Treatment* (New York: W.W. Norton, 2018), 15.

9. N. D. Volkow et al., "Cerebral Blood Flow in Chronic Cocaine Users," *British Journal of Psychiatry* 152 (May 1988): 641–48.

10. Leshner, "Addiction Is a Brain Disease," 46.

11. Erickson, *The Science of Addiction*, 72.

12. "How Addiction Hijacks the Brain," *Harvard Mental Health Letter*, July 2011, https://www.health.harvard.edu/newsletter_article/how-addiction-hijacks-the-brain.

13. Leshner, "Addiction Is a Brain Disease," 46.

14. For example, in patients such as the famous Terri Schiavo, who lived in a persistent vegetative state for more than fifteen years, fMRI scans can show that large portions of her prefrontal cortex were white (dead) matter rather than active, gray matter: "Mrs. Schiavo's brain showed global anoxic-ischemic encephalopathy resulting in massive cerebral atrophy. Her brain weight was approximately half of the expected weight. Of particular importance was the hypoxic damage and neuronal loss in her occipital lobes, which indicates cortical blindness. Her remaining brain regions show severe hypoxic injury and neuronal atrophy/loss. No areas of recent or remote traumatic injury were found." "Report of Autopsy," Medical Examiner, District Six, Pasco and Pinellas Counties, 10900 Ulmerton Road, Largo, Florida 33778. Autopsy date: April 1, 2005, p. 8.

15. "Research Finds a Single Dose of Cocaine Alters the Brain," *Birmingham News*, January 13, 2019, C-6 (story courtesy of Washington State University at Vancouver).

16. Volkow et al., "Neurobiologic Advances," 367.

17. Ronnie Cohen, "Unwise and Unnecessary: Opioids for Wisdom Teeth Extractions," *Washington Post*, March 3, 2019, https://www.washingtonpost.com/national/health-science/unwise-and-unnecessary-opioids-for-wisdom-teeth-extractions/2019/03/01/f3600a3c-2e33-11e9-86ab-5d02109aeb01_story.html?utm_term=.565de5cdbcbf (accessed July 23, 2019).

18. Gregg Caruso, *Free Will and Consciousness: A Determinist Account of the Illusion of Free Will* (Lanham, MD: Lexington Books, 2012).

19. B. Libet, C. A. Gleason, E W. Wright, and D. K. Pearl, "Time of Conscious Intention to Act in Relation to Onset of Cerebral Activity (Readiness-Potential). The Unconscious Initiation of a Freely Voluntary Act," *Brain* 106, 623–42, doi: 10.1093/brain/106.3.623; B. Libet, E. W. Wright Jr., and C. A. Gleason, "Readiness-Potentials Preceding Unrestricted 'Spontaneous' vs. Pre-planned Voluntary Acts," *Electroencephalography and Clinical Neurophysiology* 54: 322–35, doi: 10.1016/0013-4694(82)90181-X.

20. Victoria Saigle, Veljko Dubljević, and Eric Racine, "The Impact of a Landmark Neuroscience Study on Free Will: A Qualitative Analysis of Articles Using Libet and Colleagues' Methods," *American Journal of Bioethics—Neuroscience* 9, no. 1

(March 9, 2018), https://www.tandfonline.com/doi/abs/10.1080/21507740 .2018.1425756?journalCode = uabn20 (retrieved March 13, 2019).

21. Matt Shipman, "Study Tackles Neuroscience Claims to Have Disproved 'Free Will,' " *NC State News*, March 12, 2018, https://news.ncsu.edu/2018/03/free-will -review-2018/ (retrieved March 13, 2019).

22. Judy Grisel, *Never Enough: The Neuroscience and Experience of Addiction* (New York: Doubleday, 2019).

23. Judy Grisel, "The Evolutionary Advantages of an Addictive Personality," *Scientific American*, January 21, 2019, https://blogs.scientificamerican.com/observations/ the-evolutionary-advantages-of-an-addictive-personality/.

24. Grisel, "The Evolutionary Advantages."

25. Russil Durrant et al., "Drug Use and Addiction: Evolutionary Perspective," *Australian and New Zealand Journal of Psychiatry* 43 (2009): 1049–56.

26. Steve Marble, "Ronald Siegel, Drug Expert Who Believed People Naturally Like to Get High, Dies at 76," *Los Angeles Times*, April 9, 2019.

27. Ronald Siegel, *Intoxication: Life in Pursuit of Artificial Paradise* (New York: Dutton, 1989).

28. Patricia Churchland, *Conscience* (New York: W. W. Norton, 2019).

29. Adam Bisaga, *Overcoming Opioid Addiction* (New York: Experiment Publishing, 2018).

30. Harold Kincaid and Jacqueline Sullivan, "Medical Models of Addiction," in *What Is Addiction?* ed. D. Ross, H. Kincaid, D. Spurrett, and P. Collins (Cambridge, MA: MIT Press, 2010), 353–76.

31. Leshner, "Addiction Is a Brain Disease," 46.

32. Kincaid and Sullivan, "Medical Models of Addiction."

33. Sally Satel and Scott Lilienfeld, "Addiction and the Brain-Disease Fallacy," *Frontiers in Psychiatry* 4 (2013): 141, https://www.ncbi.nlm.nih.gov/pmc/articles/ PMC3939769/.

34. Herbert Fingarette, *Heavy Drinking: The Myth of Alcoholism as a Disease* (Berkeley: University of California Press, 1988), 72.

35. Harold Kincaid and Jacqueline Sullivan, "Medical Models of Addiction," in *What Is Addiction?* ed. D. Ross, H. Kincaid, D. Spurrett, and P. Collins (Cambridge, MA: MIT Press, 2010), 368.

36. Robb Stall and Patrick Biernacki, "Spontaneous Remission from the Problematic Use of Substances: An Inductive Model Derived from a Comparative Analysis of the Alcohol, Opiate, Tobacco, and Food/Obesity Literatures," *International Journal of Addictions* 21, no. 6 (1986), https://www.tandfonline.com/doi/abs/10.3109/ 10826088609063434 (retrieved March 11, 2019).

37. Satel and Lilienfled, "Addiction and the Brain-Disease Fallacy," 141.

38. Maia Szalavitz and Ryan Christopher Jones, "Addiction Doesn't Always Last a Lifetime," *New York Times*, September 1, 2018, A21.

39. Mariam Arain et al.," Maturation of the Adolescent Brain," *Neuropsychiatric*

Disease and Treatment 9 (2013): 449–61, https://www.ncbi.nlm.nih.gov/pmc/articles/PMC3621648/.

40. Jerome Kagan, *Five Constraints on Predicting Behavior* (Cambridge, MA: MIT Press, 2017), 140.

41. Kagan, *Five Constraints on Predicting Behavior*, 160.

42. Kagan, *Five Constraints on Predicting Behavior*, 163, 10 (quotes juxtaposed to make an overall point about the term *fear*).

43. Howard Markel, *An Anatomy of Addiction: Sigmund Freud, William Halsted and the Miracle Drug Cocaine* (New York: Vintage, 2011), 166.

44. The studies I examined seem to assume, or skirt, the issue of how we know a certain development of the brain corresponds to mature actions. For example, see Arain et al., "Maturation of the Adolescent Brain"; Nitin Gogtay et al., "Dynamic Mapping of Human Cortical Development during Childhood through Early Adulthood," *Proceedings of the National Academy of Sciences of United States of America* (PNAS) 101, no. 21 (May 25, 2004): 8174–79, https://doi.org/10.1073/pnas.0402680101; Jay Giedd et al., "Brain Development during Childhood and Adolescence: A Longitudinal MRI Study," *Nature Neuroscience* 2 (October 1, 1999): 861–63, https://www.nature.com/articles/nn1099_861.

CHAPTER 6

1. Jack Trimpey, *Rational Recovery: A New Cure for Substance Addiction* (New York: Simon & Schuster, 1996).

2. Immanuel Kant, "On Stupefying Oneself through Excessive Use of Food or Drink," *Metaphysics of Morals*, trans. Mary Gregor (Cambridge: Cambridge University Press, 1996; revised edition 2017), 194.

3. Immanuel Kant, "Duties towards the Body Itself," in *Lectures on Ethics*, trans. Louise Infield (Indianapolis: Hackett, 1963), 157–59.

4. Immanuel Kant, *Foundations of the Metaphysics of Morals* (1785).

5. Darren Littlejohn, *The 12-Step Buddhist: Enhance Recovery from Any Addiction* (New York: Simon & Schuster, 2009).

6. Judson Brewer, *The Craving Mind* (New Haven, CT: Yale University Press, 2017).

7. Personal accounts of overcoming heavy drinking often say the same. See Dennis Wholey, *The Courage to Change: Personal Conversation about Alcoholism* (New York: Houghton Mifflin, 1984).

8. For more on this form of (Theravada) Buddhism, see Walpola Rahula, *What the Buddha Taught: Revised and Expanded Edition with Texts from Suttas and Dhammapada* (New York: Evergreen Press, 1974).

9. Sally Satel and Scott Lilienfeld, "Addiction and the Brain-Disease Fallacy,"

Frontiers in Psychiatry 4 (2013): 141, https://www.ncbi.nlm.nih.gov/pmc/articles/PMC3939769/.

10. Louis Charland, "Decision-Making Capacity and Responsibility in Addiction," in *Addiction and Responsibility*, ed. Jeffrey Poland and George Graham (Cambridge, MA: MIT Press, 2011), 153.

11. From the cover of their book, Sally Satel and Scott Lilienfeld, *Brainwashed: The Seductive Appeal of Neuroscience* (New York: Basic Books, 2013).

12. Beverly Conyers, *Addict in the Family: Stories of Hope, Loss and Recovery, Revised and Updated* (Center City, MN: Hazelden, 2003), 12–15.

13. Laura Hilgers, "Let's Open Up about Addiction and Recovery," *New York Times*, November 5, 2017. Data cited from survey of families with addicted members by Facing Addiction.

CHAPTER 7

1. The Harm Reduction Coalition's website is http://www.harmreduction.org.

2. See the "For Smokers Only" website at http://main.uab.edu/smokersonly/show.asp?durki=63612.

3. Sanya Mansooor, "Georgia Latest State to Legalize Needle Exchange to Stop HIV," *Tuscaloosa News*, April 8, 2019, B2; Sammy Mack, "Florida Is the Latest Republican-Led State to Adopt Clean Needle Exchanges," *Tuscaloosa News*, July 8, 2019, A8.

4. Gabrielle Glasser, "Rehab Rooted in Science," *New York Times*, February 23, 2016, D4.

5. Quoted in Richardo Alonso-Zaldivar and Carla K. Johnson, "The New War on Drugs," *Birmingham News*, February 3, 2019.

6. Dr. DeLuca's professional website is http://www.doctordeluca.com/.

7. Brad Rodu, *For Smokers Only: How Smokeless Tobacco Can Save Your Life* (Hermosa Beach, CA: Sumner Books, 2016).

8. Ricardo Alonso-Saldivar, "Plan to Stop HIV Epidemic Targets High-Infection Areas," *Tuscaloosa News*, February 9, 2019, B3.

9. "Ending the HIV Epidemic," HIV.gov, https://www.hiv.gov/federal-response/ending-the-hiv-epidemic/overview (accessed May 18, 2019).

10. Cited by Colton Wooten, "Quitting Heroin in the Sunshine State," *New York Times*, March 15, 2018, D1, 4.

11. CDC, "Alcohol-Impaired Driving," https://www.cdc.gov/motorvehiclesafety/pdf/PolicyImpact-Alcohol-a.pdf (accessed February 5, 2019).

12. CDC, "Alcohol-Impaired Driving."

13. Leslie Jamison, *The Recovering: Intoxication and Its Aftermath* (New York: Little, Brown, 2018), 449.

14. See Jamison, *The Recovering*, 450.

15. "Understanding Naloxone," Harm Reduction Coalition, https://harmreduc tion.org/issues/overdose-prevention/overview/overdose-basics/understanding -naloxone/ (accessed May 18, 2019).

16. Scott Shackford, "Harm Reduction Is Helping Reduce Ohio Opioid Over-dose Deaths," *Reason*, December 18, 2018.

17. Abby Goodnough, "This City's Overdose Deaths Have Plunged. Can Others Learn from It?" *New York Times*, November 25, 2018.

18. Barbara Ostrov, "More States Say Doctors Must Offer Overdose Reversal Drug," *Kaiser Health News*, February 19, 2019.

19. Martha Bebinger, "Nurse Denied Life Insurance Because She Carries Nalox-one," National Public Radio, December 13, 2018, https://www.npr.org/sections/ health-shots/2018/12/13/674586548/nurse-denied-life-insurance-because-she -carries-naloxone (accessed February 10, 2019).

20. Camille Bains, "New Opioid Treatment," *Global News*, March 4, 2019.

21. Isabela Kwai, "An Australian Doctor's Dream: Curing America's Opioid Cri-sis," *New York Times*, June 7, 2019, A7.

22. Kim Painter, "Hope and Help amid Opioid OD Epidemic," *USA Today*, January 22, 2019, A2.

23. "Vermont Opioid Related Fatalities," Vermont Department of Public Health, http://www.healthvermont.gov/sites/default/files/documents/pdf/ADAP_ Data_Brief_Opioid_Related_Fatalities.pdf (accessed May 18, 2019).

24. Painter, "Hope and Help amid Opioid OD Epidemic."

25. "Supervised Drug Consumption: Evidence-Based Public Health," Harm Reduction Coalition, https://harmreduction.org/blog/sif_dcr/ (accessed January 20, 2019).

26. King County Heroin and Prescription Opiate Addiction Task Force, https:// www.kingcounty.gov/~/media/depts/community-human-services/behavioral-health/ documents/herointf/Final-Heroin-Opiate-Addiction-Task-_Force-Report.ashx ?la=en (accessed January 29, 2019).

27. Harm Reduction Coalition, *Alternatives to Public Injection*, 2016, https:// harmreduction.org/wp-content/uploads/2016/05/Alternatives-to-Public-Injection -report.pdf.

28. Claudia Stoicescu and Catherine Cook, *Harm Reduction in Europe: Mapping Coverage and Civil Society Advocacy*, European Harm Reduction Network, 15, https:// www.hri.global/files/2011/12/20/EHRN_CivilSocietyCompiled_WebFinal.pdf (accessed March 13, 2019).

29. "'Dozens and Dozens' of Underground Safe Injection Sites in Seattle," *My Northwest*, November 18, 2017, https://mynorthwest.com/1167554/seattle-under ground-safe-injection-sites/ (accessed July 23, 2019).

30. Matt Driscoll, "From 13,000 Tacoma to 100 Million Nationwide, Needle Exchange Program Proves Worth Over 30 Years," *Tacoma News Tribune*, September 14, 2018, https://www.thenewstribune.com/news/local/news-columns-blogs/matt -driscoll/article218298450.html.

31. Casey Leins, "New Hampshire: Ground Zero for Opioids," *US News and World Report*, June 28, 2017.

32. Tim Lahey, "Let Opioid Users Inject in Hospitals," *New York Times*, January 6, 2017, A19, https://www.drugabuse.gov/drugs-abuse/opioids/opioid-summaries-by -state.

33. Jennifer Percy, "Trapped by the 'Walmart of Heroin,' " *New York Times*, October 10, 2018, https://www.nytimes.com/2018/10/10/magazine/kensington-heroin -opioid-philadelphia.html (accessed January 23, 2019).

34. Abby Goodnough, "U.S. Sues to Stop Safe Site for Users of Illicit Opioids," *New York Times*, February 7, 2019, A15.

35. Rod Rosenstein, "The Dangers of 'Safe Injection,' " *New York Times*, September 29, 2018, A19.

36. Percy, "Trapped by the 'Walmart of Heroin.' "

37. Stephanie Knoll, "The US Can Learn a Lot from Zurich about How to Fight Its Heroin Crisis," *PRI*, February 12, 2016, https://www.pri.org/stories/2016-02-12/ us-can-learn-lot-zurich-about-how-fight-its-heroin-crisis (accessed January 23, 2019).

38. Gerald W. Lynch and Roberta Blotner, "The Case for Decriminalizing Drugs Dies in Zurich," *New York Times*, letter, March 13, 1992.

39. Arnold Trebach, President, Drug Policy Foundation, "Why Zurich's Bad Idea on Drugs Went Wrong," *New York Times*, March 27, 1992.

40. "Insite," Wikipedia, https://en.wikipedia.org/wiki/Insite.

41. Ecstasy, or "Molly," is methylendediozymethamphatamine, or MDMA. MDA, or "Sally," is methylenedioxyamphetamine, thought by some users to give a smoother, gentler high than Molly. However, some users report that MDA is more stimulating, longer lasting, and more potent than MDMA, and Sally has been involved in overdose deaths. Sassafras oil contains safrole, which can be used to make either MDMA or MDA. "What Is Sassafras?" Recovery First, February 11, 2009, https://www.recovery-first.org/drug-abuse/what-is-sassafras/; Andrea Woo, "Family of Girl Who Fatally Overdoses Pushes for Drug Check Expansion," *The Globe and Mail* (Vancouver), April 20, 2019; Evan Wood, "Strategies for Reducing Opioid-Overdose Deaths—Lessons from Canada," *New England Journal of Medicine* 378, no. 17 (April 26, 2018): 1565–67.

42. I owe this point to Dave Kummerlowe and his CADRE company.

43. Nicholas Kristoff, "How to Win the War on Drugs," *New York Times*, September 24, 2017, 1.

44. Michael Farell et al., *Reviewing Current Practice in Drug-Substitution Treatment in the European Union* (Lisbon: EMCDDA, 2000), http://www.emcdda.europa .eu/attachements.cfm/att_33997_EN_Insight3.pdf.

45. Kristoff, "How to Win the War on Drugs," 2.

46. "Did Portugal Really Legalize All Drugs?" Narconon, May 13, 2018, https:// www.narconon.org/blog/did-portugal-really-legalize-all-drugs.html (accessed May 18, 2019).

47. Jen Gunter, "Drinking while Pregnant: An Inconvenient Truth," *New York Times*, February 5, 2019, https://www.nytimes.com/2019/02/05/style/drinking-while-pregnant.html?smid=nytcore-ios-share.

48. Phillip May et al., "Prevalence of Fetal Alcohol Spectrum Disorders in 4 US Communities," *Journal of the American Medical Association* 319, no. 5 (February 6, 2018): 474–82, https://jamanetwork.com/journals/jama/fullarticle/2671465.

49. "Breastfeeding and Alcohol," Centers for Disease Control, https://www.cdc .gov/breastfeeding/breastfeeding-special-circumstances/vaccinations-medications -drugs/alcohol.html (accessed April 10, 2019).

50. "However, opioid addicts have been compared to their own nonaddicted siblings to examine exposure to intrapartum analgesics documented decades earlier in their birth records. Infants who became opioid addicts had nearly five times the exposure to maternal analgesics than their nonaddicted siblings, and there was a dose-response with increasing addiction risk seen with increased obstetric drug exposure. Similar work has suggested that human adult amphetamine addiction is similarly influenced by early-life, peripartum maternal analgesic exposure. While these studies examined intra-partum rather than lactation-induced opioid exposure to the baby, they nonetheless provide evidence of lifelong risk conferred by brief, early-life, opioid exposure. Thus, the real concern is not whether breast fed infants of opioid consuming mothers will be at risk of respiratory depression, but to what extent they may be at risk of life-long, subtle, alterations in cognitive, emotional, and motivational function. We should be honest with our patients that in these domains these drugs are not known to be safe, and we have substantial reason to believe they are not safe. Every effort should be made to limit infant exposure to opioids through breast milk. Chronic opioid use, in particular, among breast feeding mothers should be assumed to be unsafe for the developing mind of the infant until further data suggests otherwise." Ian R. Carroll, "Opioids and Lactation: Insufficient Evidence of Safety," *Pain Medicine* 16, no. 4 (April 2015): 628–30.

51. Maia Szalavitz, "When the Cure Is Worse Than the Disease," *New York Times*, February 20, 2019, SR6.

52. Travis Rieder, *In Pain: A Bioethicist's Personal Struggle with Opioids* (New York: HarperCollins, 2019).

CHAPTER 8

1. "Genetics of Alcohol Use Disorder," National Institute on Alcohol Abuse and Alcoholism, https://www.niaaa.nih.gov/alcohol-health/overview-alcohol-consumption/ alcohol-use-disorders/genetics-alcohol-use-disorders (accessed January 23, 2019).

2. Gabrielle Glasser, "Rehab Rooted in Science," *New York Times*, February 23, 2016, D4.

3. Shalini Ramachandran, Zolan Kanno-Youngs, and Yoree Koh, "The Rise and Fall of a Tech Genius," *Wall Street Journal*, February 16, 2019.

4. Paul Thomas and Jennifer Margulis, *The Addiction Spectrum: A Compassionate, Holistic Model to Recovery* (New York: HarperCollins, 2018), 46.

5. Thomas and Margulis, *The Addiction Spectrum*, 1.

6. Thomas and Margulis, *The Addiction Spectrum*, 47.

7. Caroline Hallemann, "How Donald Trump's Brother Fred Jr. Shaped His Views on Addiction," *Town & Country*, October 26, 2017, https://www.townandcountry mag.com/society/politics/a13098008/fred-trump-jr-addiction-history/ (accessed July 23, 2019).

8. "Why Alcoholism Runs in Families," Recovery Village, https://www.therecovery village.com/alcohol-abuse/faq/alcoholism-runs-families/#gref.

9. L. Bevilacqua and D. Goldman, "Genes and Addictions," *Clinical Pharmacology and Therapeutics* 85, no. 4 (April 2009): 359–61.

10. Bevilacqua and Goldman, "Genes and Addictions."

11. Robert Morse, MD, quoted in "Does Addiction Run in Families? What Statistics Reveal," Recovery Center, https://www.orlandorecovery.com/blog/does-addic tion-run-in-families-addiction-in-families-statistics/#gref (accessed January 24, 2019).

12. National Institute on Alcohol Abuse and Alcoholism, https://www.niaaa.nih .gov/research/major-initiatives/collaborative-studies-genetics-alcoholism-coga-study.

13. Carlton Erickson, *The Science of Addiction: From Neurobiology to Treatment* (New York: W.W. Norton, 2018), 72.

14. J. R. Minkel, "'Methuselah' Mutation Linked to Longer Life," *Scientific American*, March 4, 2008.

15. Cormac O'Brien, *The Forgotten History of America* (New York: Crestline Books, 2018).

16. Renee C. Fox and Judith P. Swazey, *The Courage to Fail: A Social View of Organ Transplants and Dialysis* (New York: Routledge, 2017), 300.

17. Lawrence K. Altman, "Artificial Kidney Use Poses Awesome Questions," *New York Times*, October 23, 1971. Quoted in Fox and Swazey, *The Courage to Fail*, 266.

18. Connie Mulligan et al., "Allelic Variation at Alcohol Metabolism Genes (ADH1B, ALDH1C, ALDH2) and Alcohol Dependence in Native Americans," *Human Genetics* 113 (July 12, 2003): 325–36.

19. D. W. Crabb, M. Matsumoto, D. Chang, and M. You, "Overview of the Role of Alcohol Dehydrogenase and Aldehyde Dehydrogenase and Their Variants in the Genesis of Alcohol-related Pathology," *Proceedings of the Nutritional Society* 63, no. 1 (February 2004): 49–63.

20. E. Quertemont, "Genetic Polymorphism in Ethanol Metabolism: Acetaldehyde Contribution to Alcohol Abuse and Alcoholism," *Molecular Psychiatry* 9, no. 6 (June 004): 570–81.

21. Thanks to Stephen Austad of the UAB biology department for helping me clarify how this process works.

22. A switch of a base in DNA of ALDH2 gene leads to ALDH2*2 enzyme, which has less than 15 percent of the activity needed to neutralize acetaldehyde.

23. H. J. Edenberg, "The Genetics of Alcohol Metabolism: Role of Alcohol Dehydrogenase and Aldehyde Dehydrogenase Variants," *Alcohol Research Health* 30, no. 1 (2007): 5–13, https://www.ncbi.nlm.nih.gov/pmc/articles/PMC3860432/.

24. "Profile, Dr. Cindy Ehlers," National Institute on Alcohol Abuse and Alcoholism, https://pubs.niaaa.nih.gov/publications/healthdisparities/profile.html.

25. Ibid.

26. Cindy Ehlers and Ian Gizer, "Evidence for a Genetic Component for Substance Dependence in Native Americans," *American Journal of Psychiatry* 170, no. 2 (February 2013), https://ajp.psychiatryonline.org/doi/pdf/10.1176/appi.ajp .2012.12010113.

27. Ibid., from the abstract.

28. Roxanne Dunbar-Ortiz and Dina Gilio-Whitaker, "What's Behind the Myth of Native American Alcoholism?" *Pacific Standard*, October 10, 2016, https://psmag .com/news/whats-behind-the-myth-of-native-american-alcoholism (accessed April 12, 2019).

29. Carl Zimmer, "The Famine Ended 70 Years Ago, but Dutch Genes Still Bear Scars," *New York Times*, January 31, 2018.

30. Bailey Kirkpatrick, "Dad's Drinking Could Epigenetically Affect Son's Sensitivity and Preference for Alcohol," What Is Epigenetics, June 18, 2014, https://www .whatisepigenetics.com/dads-drinking-could-epigenetically-affect-sons-sensitivity-and -preference-for-alcohol/.

31. "Genetics of Alcohol Use Disorder," National Institute on Alcohol Abuse and Alcoholism, https://www.niaaa.nih.gov/alcohol-health/overview-alcohol-consumption/ alcohol-use-disorders/genetics-alcohol-use-disorders.

32. "What Is It about Chronic Pain?" Science of Addiction, *Family Parade Magazine*, March 2019, 16.

33. Katie Hunt, "Woman Who Feels No Pain Could Help Scientists Develop New Painkillers," CBS News, March 28, 2019, https://www.cnn.com/2019/03/28/ health/woman-feels-no-pain-gene-mutation/index.html.

34. D. Goldman, G. Oroszi, and F. Ducci, "The Genetics of Addiction: Uncovering the Genes," *National Review of Genetics* 6 (2005): 521–32.

35. A. Agrawal et al., "The Genetics of Addiction—a Translational Perspective," *Translational Psychiatry* 2 (2012): e140.

36. Henri Begleiter and B. Poriesz, "What Is Inherited in the Disposition toward Alcoholism? A Proposed Model," *Alcoholism: Clinical and Experimental Research* 7 (July 23, 1999): 1125–35, https://doi.org/10.1111/j.1530-0277.1999.tb04269.x (accessed February 6, 2019).

37. Rachel Torres et al., "Traditional Practices, Traditional Spirituality, and Alcohol Cessation among American Indians," *Journal of Studies on Alcohol* 67, no. 2 (2006): 236–44, https://www.jsad.com/doi/abs/10.15288/jsa.2006.67.236.

38. Mulligan et al., "Allelic Variation at Alcohol Metabolism Genes."

39. Sherman Alexie, *You Don't Have to Say You Love Me: A Memoir* (New York: Little, Brown, 2017), 19.

40. Bevilacqua and Goldman, "Genes and Addictions."

41. Herbert Fingarette, "Why We Should Reject the Disease Concept of Alcoholism," in *Controversies in the Addiction Field*, ed. Ruth C. Engs (Dububuqe, IA: Kendall-Hunt, 1990).

CHAPTER 9

1. Nora Volkow et al., "Neurobiologic Advances from the Brain Model of Addiction," *New England Journal of Medicine* 374 (2016): 363–71.

2. March Lewis, "Brain Change in Addiction as Learning, Not Disease," *New England Journal of Medicine* 379, no. 16 (2018): 1551–60.

3. Marc Lewis, *The Biology of Desire: Why Addiction Is Not a Disease* (New York: Public Affairs, 2016).

4. Maia Szalavitz, *Unbroken Brain: A Revolutionary Way of Understanding Addiction* (New York: Picador, 2016), 2.

5. Sally Satel and Scott Lilienfeld, "Addiction and the Brain-Disease Fallacy," *Frontiers in Psychiatry* 4 (2013): 141, https://www.ncbi.nlm.nih.gov/pmc/articles/PMC3939769/.

6. Maia Szalavitz, "When the Cure Is Worse Than the Disease," *New York Times*, February 9, 2019.

7. Szalavitz, *Unbroken Brain*, 6.

8. Maia Szalavitz, *Help at Any Cost: How the Troubled-Teen Industry Cons Parents and Hurts Kids* (New York: Riverhead Books, 2006).

9. Szalavitz, *Unbroken Brain*, 3.

10. Szalavitz, *Unbroken Brain*, 4.

11. Mariam Arain et al., "Maturation of the Adolescent Brain," *Neuropsychiatric Disease and Treatment* 9 (2013): 449–61, https://www.ncbi.nlm.nih.gov/pmc/articles/PMC3621648/.

12. Szalawitz, *Unbroken Brain*, 176.

13. Owen Flanagan, "What Is It Like to Be an Addict?" in *Addiction and Responsibility*, ed. Jeffrey Poland and George Graham (Cambridge, MA: MIT Press, 2011), 269–92.

14. Stanly Milgram, *Obedience to Authority* (New York: Harper & Row, 1974).

15. Timothy McMahan King, "Even Heroes Can Struggle with Addiction," *Wall Street Journal*, July 12, 2019, https://www.wsj.com/articles/even-heroes-can-struggle-with-addiction-11562969041 (accessed July 23, 2019).

16. This situation occurs in suburbs of Birmingham, Alabama, and was described

to me by a long-practicing psychiatrist at UAB Hospitals. I know the practicing physicians involved in running these groups.

17. Jack Trimpey, *Rational Recovery: The New Cure for Substance Addiction: The Revolutionary Alternative to Alcoholics Anonymous* (New York: Pocket Books, 1996), 70.

18. R. J. Solberg, *The Dry Drunk Syndrome* (Center City, MN: Hazelden, 1983).

19. Terence Gorski, *Staying Sober: A Guide to Relapse Prevention* (Independence, MO: Independence Press, 1986); Denis Daley and Antoine Douailhy, *Relapse Prevention Counseling: Clinical Strategies to Guide Addiction Recovery and Reduce Relapse* (Eau Claire, WI: PESI Publishing & Media, 2015).

20. Trimpey, *Rational Recovery*.

CHAPTER 10

1. David Itzkoff, *Robin* (New York: Henry Holt, 2018) 345.

2. Paco is the popular name for the distillation of a cocaine paste made from the coca leaf, which can contain as much as 90 percent cocaine sulfate. In Brazil, it is cheap and commonly smoked with tobacco or pot by poor workers to boost energy.

3. John Rawls, *A Theory of Justice* (Cambridge, MA: Harvard University Press, 1973).

4. A. Maddison, *Contours of the World Economy I—2030 AD* (Oxford: Oxford University Press, 2007), 194.

5. Thomas Hager, *Ten Drugs: How Plants, Powders, and Pills Have Shaped the History of Medicine* (New York: Abrams, 2019).

6. George Will, "Worse Living through Chemistry," *Tuscaloosa News*, March 17, 2019, A11, quoting the *Financial Times*.

7. Will, "Worse Living through Chemistry."

8. Don Winslow, *The Power of the Dog, the Cartel, the Border* (New York: William Morrow, 2019).

9. For example, see Joseph Stiglitz's *The Great Divide: Unequal Societies and What We Can Do about Them* (New York: W. W. Norton, 2015); Nancy Isenberg, *White Trash: The 400-Year Untold History of Class in America* (New York: Viking, 2016).

10. "Opioid Deaths by State," National Institute on Drug and Alcohol Abuse, https://www.drugabuse.gov/drugs-abuse/opioids/opioid-summaries-by-state (accessed May 18, 2019).

11. Taylor Stuck, "West Virginia's Poverty Rate Increases to 19.1 Percent," *Herald-Dispatch*, September 14, 2018.

12. JoAnn Snoderly, "West Virginia Again Leads Nation in Drug Overdose Deaths," *Exponent Telegram* (Clarksburg, WV), November 29, 2018.

13. Lindsey Bever, "A Town of 3200 Was Flooded with Nearly 21 Million Pain

Pills as Addiction Crisis Worsened, Lawmakers Say," *Washington Post*, January 31, 2018.

14. Jan Hoffman, Katie Thomas, and Danny Hakim, "3,271 Pill Bottles, a Town of 2,831: Court Filings Say Corporations Fed Opioid Epidemic," *New York Times*, July 23, 2019 (accessed July 23, 2019).

15. Curt Anderson, "Hooked, Hoodwinked: Some Drug Rehabs Aim for Relapse," *Tuscaloosa News*, August 25, 2017, A4.

16. Anderson, "Hooked, Hoodwinked."

17. Victor Fuchs, *Who Shall Live? Health, Economics, and Social Choice* (Hackensack, NJ: World Scientific Publishing, 2011).

18. Ryan Christopher Jones, "How Photography Exploits the Vulnerable," *New York Times*, August 31, 2018.

19. Shaila Dewan, "A Growing Chorus of Big City Prosecutors Say No to Marijuana Convictions," *New York Times*, January 30, 2019, x.

20. Trip Gabriel, "2020 Democrats Find Common Cause in Pot," *New York Times*, March 18, 2010, A10.

21. Abdullah Shihipar, "The Opioid Crisis Isn't White," *New York Times*, February 27, 2019, A25.

22. US Bureau of Justice Statistics, "Prisoners in 2016," updated August 7, 2018, https://www.bjs.gov/content/pub/pdf/p16.pdf.

23. Hager, *Ten Drugs*.

24. I. A. Binswager et al., "Release from Prison—A High Risk of Death of Former Inmates," *New England Journal of Medicine* 356 (2007): 157–65.

25. Ingrid Binswager, "Opioid Use Disorder and Incarceration—Hope for Ensuring the Continuity of Treatment," *New England Journal of Medicine* 380 (March 28, 2019): 1193–95.

26. Even an arrest, not a conviction, for drugs from fifty years ago can prevent one from getting entry back into the United States from abroad when traveling.

27. F. J. Freyer, "Court Orders Essex County to Provide Methadone to Inmate," *Boston Globe*, November 27, 2018, https://www.bostonglobe.com/metro/2018/11/27/court-orders-essex-county-provide-methadone-inmate/iz5GxxfwgKPmi5CNWtNrnK/story.html.

28. Abby Goodnough, "Woman Sues US Prison System Over Ban on Methadone to Treat Drug Addiction," *New York Times*, March 16, 2019, A21.

29. Michael Bloomberg, "Ending the Opioid Crisis in Seven Steps," *Tuscaloosa News*, January 14, 2019.

30. "Feds Still Aren't up to Dealing with Opioid Crisis, So We're Stepping In: Bloomberg & Wolf," *USA Today*, November 13, 2018, https://www.usatoday.com/story/opinion/2018/11/30/michael-bloomberg-tom-wolf-opioid-crisis-donation-pennsylvania-overdose-column/2151012002/.

31. Nicholas Kristoff, "How to Win the War on Drugs," *New York Times*, September 24, 2017, 1.

32. Centers for Disease Control, "During Binges, U.S. Adults Have 17 Billion Drinks a Year," press release, March 16, 2018, https://www.cdc.gov/media/releases/2018/p0316-binge-drinking.html (Retrieved February 4, 2019).

33. Hilary Aroke et al., "Estimating the Direct Costs of Outpatient Opioid Prescriptions: A Retrospective Analysis of Data from the Rhode Island Prescription Drug Monitoring Program," *Journal of Managed Care & Specialty Pharmacy* 24, no. 3 (March 2018): 214–24.

34. Statisica, "Prescription Drug Expenditure in the United States from 1960 to 2018 (in Billion U.S. Dollars)," *The Statistics Portal*, https://www.statista.com/statistics/184914/prescription-drug-expenditures-in-the-us-since-1960/ (accessed February 4, 2019).

35. World Health Organization, "Alcohol Consumers by Country," Global Health Observatory Data Repository, http://apps.who.int/gho/data/node.main.A1044?lang=en (accessed March 11, 2019).

36. Petula Dvorak, "With Her Axe, She Carved a Path to Prohibition a Century Ago," *Washington Post*, January 16, 2019.

37. Public Citizen, quoted by Carl Elliott, "The Drug Pushers," *Atlantic*, April 2006, https://www.theatlantic.com/magazine/archive/2006/04/the-drug-pushers/304714/ (accessed February 3, 2019).

38. Carl Elliott, *White Coat, Black Hat: Adventures on the Dark Side of Medicine* (Boston: Beacon Press, 2011).

39. "Two months before resigning as chair of the U.S. House Committee on Energy and Commerce, which oversees the drug industry, Tauzin had played a key role in shepherding through Congress the Medicare Prescription Drug Bill. Democrats said that the bill was 'a give-away to the drugmakers' because it prohibits the government from negotiating lower drug prices and bans the importation of identical, cheaper, drugs from Canada and elsewhere. The Veterans Affairs agency, which can negotiate drug prices, pays much less than Medicare does. The bill was passed in an unusual congressional session at 3 a.m. under heavy pressure from the drug companies" (see https://en.wikipedia.org/wiki/Billy_Tauzin).

40. The Koch brothers often fund such studies, for example, at the Institute for Humane Studies at George Mason University or the business school at Troy State University in Alabama, as well as at many other universities.

41. Jack Trimpey, *Rational Recovery: A New Cure for Substance Addiction* (New York: Simon & Schuster, 1996).

42. Tom Metcalf and Simon Kennedy, "Davos Billionaires Keep Getting Richer: The World's Elite Have Prospered since the Financial Crash," *Bloomberg News*, January 19, 2019, https://www.bloomberg.com/news/articles/2019-01-20/dimon-schwarzman-and-other-davos-a-listers-add-175-billion-in-10-years.

43. Jamie Ducharme and Elijah Wolfson, "Does ZIP Code Equal Life Expectancy?" *Time*, July 8, 2019, 8.

44. Of course, a single person would need at least $1,000 a month for a studio

apartment there, so a gross income per month of at least $2,500 month or $30,000 a year, which would require a decent job, which would likely come with medical coverage. For a single parent, it would be harder, probably requiring a one-bedroom apartment and more money for day care or after-school care.

CHAPTER 11

1. Glenn A. Case, Sandra Distefano, and Barry K. Logant, "Tabulation of Alcohol Content of Beer and Malt Beverages," *Journal of Analytical Toxology* 24, no. 3 (April 2000): 201–10.

2. Greg Bishop, "An NFL Star and His Marijuana Journey," in *Marijuana: The Medical Movement* (*Time* magazine special edition), April 2019, 32.

3. Jeffrey Kluger, "Some Words of Caution," in *Marijuana: The Medical Movement* (*Time* magazine special edition), April 2019, 62.

4. Yasmin Hurd of Mt. Sinai Hospital, quoted in Kluger, "Some Words of Caution," 63.

5. My EMSAP research assistant, Melissa Ebling, did most of the research for this section.

6. American Academy of Pediatrics, "American Academy of Pediatrics Reaffirms Opposition to Legalizing Marijuana for Recreational or Medical Use," January 26, 2015, https://www.aap.org/en-us/about-the-aap/aap-press-room/Pages/American-Academy-of-Pediatrics-Reaffirms-Opposition-to-Legalizing-Marijuana-for-Recreational-or-Medical-Use.aspx.

7. Kenneth L. Davis and Mary Jeanne Kreek, "Marijuana Damages Young Brains," *New York Times*, June 17, 2019, A19.

8. American Academy of Pediatrics, "The Impact of Marijuana Policies on Youth: Clinical, Research, and Legal Update," *Pediatrics* 135, no. 3 (March 2015): 584–87.

9. "Is Vaping a Gateway Drug?" Keck School of Medicine Blog, https://www.keckmedicine.org/is-vaping-a-gateway-drug/; "Vaping—The New Gateway to Drug Addiction," talk by Susan Walley, MD, assistant professor of pediatrics, Children's Hospital of Alabama, September 20, 2019, Community Breakfast for Freedom from Addiction Coalition, Birmingham, Alabama.

10. Nadia Kounang and Michael Nedelman, "North Carolina Sues Juul, Claiming Deceptive Marketing and Targeting Youth," CNN, May 15, 2009, https://www.cnn.com/2019/05/15/health/north-carolina-juul-lawsuit-bn/index.html.

11. George Will, "The Puzzling Problem of Vaping," *Tuscaloosa News*, July 21, 2019, A15.

12. Centers for Disease Control, "Outbreak of Lung Injury Associated with E-Cigarette Use, or Vaping," https://www.cdc.gov/tobacco/basic_information/e-cigarettes/severe-lung-disease.html. This figure comes from the CDC in October 2019. By November 5, 2019, the number of deaths had risen to thirty-nine.

13. Jason Mudd, "Get Company Ready for the Hemp Age," *Birmingham Business Journal*, March 15, 2019, 11, https://www.brightfieldgroup.com.

14. "CBD: On a Real Market High," CBS News, May 5, 2019, https://www.cbsnews.com/news/cbd-on-a-real-market-high-swiftly-growing-demand-for-cannabidiol-products/.

15. Malcolm Gladwell, "Unwatched Pot: Do We Know Enough about Marijuana?" *The New Yorker*, January 14, 2019.

16. L. Borgelt et al., "The Pharmacologic and Clinical Effects of Medical Cannabis," *Pharmacotherapy* 33, no. 2 (2013), 205.

17. Jayne O'Donnell et al., "High Risks: As Marijuana Gains Acceptance, Opponents Point to Its Dark Side," *USA Today*, March 11, 2019.

18. Kate Taylor, "Skeptical of Legalizing Pot Amid Opioid Crisis," *New York Times*, February 21, 2019, 18.

19. Taylor, "Skeptical of Legalizing Pot."

20. Jonathan Lieberson, "The Reality of AIDS," *New York Review of Books*, January 16, 1986.

21. Lindsey Tanner, "Marijuana Use Doubles in US Pregnant Woman to 1 in 14," *Tuscaloosa News*, June 19, 2019, A5.

CHAPTER 12

1. Julia Philips, *You'll Never Eat Lunch in This Town Again* (New York: Random House, 1991).

2. Scott Higham, Sari Horwitz, and Steven Rich, "76 Billion Opioid Pills: Newly Released Federal Data Unmasks the Epidemic," *Washington Post*, July 16, 2019, https://www.washingtonpost.com/investigations/76-billion-opioid-pills-newly-released-federal-data-unmasks-the-epidemic/2019/07/16/5f29fd62-a73e-11e9-86dd-d7f0e60391e9_story.html?utm_term = .b275ef4a3c18.

3. Higham et al., "76 Billion Opioid Pills."

4. Geogg Mulvihill and Riin Aljaas, "Even as the Nation's Opioid Crisis Grew, the Pills Got Stronger," *Tuscaloosa News*, July 25, 2019, A4.

5. Keith Humphreys, "We Can't Fight Opioids by Controlling Demand Alone," *Washington Post*, July 5, 2019, https://www.washingtonpost.com/outlook/we-cant-fight-opioids-by-controlling-demand-alone/2019/07/05/d025358e-7e2d-11e9-8ede-f4abf521ef17_story.html?utm_term = .4e87f7b4e3e1.

INDEX

ABOUT THE AUTHOR

Gregory E. Pence has taught bioethics to medical and premedical students for forty-four years at the University of Alabama at Birmingham (UAB). His other works in bioethics include a bestselling textbook and seven trade books. In 2019 at UAB, partly because of this book, he won the Ireland Award for Scholarly Distinction.